OXFORD MEDICAL PUBLICATIONS

Health Promotion for Pharmacists

Health Promotion for Pharmacists

Second edition

Alison Blenkinsopp
PhD, BPharm, MRPharmS

Professor of the Practice of Pharmacy,
Department of Medicines Management, Keele University

Rhona Panton
MPhil, MRPharmS

Non-Executive Director, Worcester Community Trust

Claire Anderson
PhD, BSc, MRPharmS

Director of Pharmacy Practice and Social Pharmacy,
The Pharmacy School, University of Nottingham

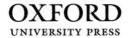
OXFORD
UNIVERSITY PRESS

Bib : 37311

OXFORD
UNIVERSITY PRESS

Great Clarendon Street, Oxford OX2 6DP

Oxford University Press is a department of the University of Oxford.
It furthers the University's objectives of excellence in research, scholarship,
and education by publishing worldwide in

Oxford New York
Athens Auckland Bangkok Bogotá Buenos Aires Calcutta
Cape Town Chennai Dar es Salaam Delhi Florence Hong Kong Istanbul
Karachi Kuala Lumpur Madrid Melbourne Mexico City Mumbai
Nairobi Paris São Paulo Singapore Taipei Tokyo Toronto Warsaw
and associated companies in Berlin Ibadan

Oxford is a registered trade mark of Oxford University Press
in the UK and in certain other countries

Published in the United States
by Oxford University Press, Inc., New York

British Library Cataloguing in Publication Data
Data available

Library of Congress Cataloging in Publication Data
Blenkinsopp, Alison.
Health promotion for pharmacists / Alison Blenkinsopp, Rhona
Panton, Claire Anderson. – 2nd ed.
(Oxford medical publications)
Includes bibliographical references and index.
1. Pharmacist and patient. 2. Health promotion. I. Panton,
Rhona. II. Anderson, Claire, PhD. III. Title. IV. Series.
[DNLM: 1. Health Promotion. 2. Health Behavior.
3. Pharmaceutical Services. 4. Primary Prevention. 5. Risk
Factors. WA 108 B647h 2000]
RS56.B57   2000   613'.024'615–dc21   99-40698

1 3 5 7 9 10 8 6 4 2

ISBN 0 19 263044 X

Typset by Downdell, Oxford
Printed in Great Britain
on acid-free paper by
Biddles Ltd,
Guildford & King's Lynn

Preface to the Second Edition

Since the first edition of this book was completed in 1991 the pharmacist's role in health promotion has become more widely recognized. Here, in the second edition, we have of course updated relevant material and have added new chapters. The new material incorporates the changes in the evidence base for health promotion and sets the context of health care policy to show how pharmacists can contribute to public health over the next decade.

The book has three sections. In the first (Chapters 1 to 3) we cover the background to health promotion, health policy and the major health challenges facing society. The second section (Chapters 4 to 6) considers behaviour and how it can be changed, the development of health promotion in pharmacy, and the role of medicines in promoting health.

The third section of the book addresses specific health promotion topics (Chapters 7 to 15), all of which have been updated and substantially rewritten. Case studies and practical examples are included throughout the book together with possible approaches the pharmacist might take. Each chapter has been reviewed by an expert in the field to ensure its currency and relevance to practice.

We hope the book will inspire you to develop your own professional practice in health promotion and provide a supply of ideas for working with others in this important field.

August 1999.   AB, RP, CA

Acknowledgements

We would like to thank all the experts who reviewed individual chapters and contributed additional ideas. They were:

Chapters 1 & 2   Jane Todd, Health Promotion Specialist, Harpenden.

Chapter 3   Colette McCreedy, Head of Practice Division, National Pharmaceutical Association.

Chapters 4 & 5   Nikki Davey, Specialist Pharmacist, Southampton.

Chapter 6   Dr. Theo Raynor, Head of Division of Academic Pharmacy Practice, University of Leeds.

Chapter 7   Dr. Hazel Sinclair, Department of General Practice, University of Aberdeen.

Chapter 8   Dr. Pamela Mason, Pharmaceutical Consultant and Writer, London.

Chapter 9   Dr. Adrian Taylor Senior Lecturer in Exercise and Health Physiology, University of Brighton.

Chapter 10   Professor Andy Blinkhorn, Department of Oral Health & Development, Turner Dental School, University of Manchester.

Chapter 11   Tony Belfield, Director of Information, fpa, London.

Chapter 12   Dr. Sarah Jarvis, General Practitioner and Medical Writer, London.

Chapter 13   Dr. Eileen Scott, School of Pharamcy, Queen's University of Belfast.

Ron Morley assisted with word-processing of the manuscript.

Contents

To John and Howard

1 What is health promotion?

When asked to identify those factors which have made the greatest impact on health in the UK in the last century, many pharmacists, like other health professionals, will cite the introduction of vaccination programmes and the discovery of antibiotics. In fact, the reduction of mortality from the major killer diseases of the nineteenth and early twentieth century began long before the advent of either vaccination or antibiotics.

The factors which played the largest part in improving health were societal changes, particularly the introduction of legislation to improve living conditions and sanitation, and the creation of the Welfare State.

This chapter will review the history of the changing health of the population since the mid- nineteenth century and will address some of the key issues in health promotion today. The social, political, personal, and medical factors which influence our health will be discussed. This background is essential for pharmacists to understand the context of the health promotion activities and advice which they might offer.

1.1 What is health?

Health means different things to different people and many attempts have been made to define it. Health is:

A state of complete physical, mental and social well-being and not merely the absence of disease or infirmity (World Health Organization (WHO), 1947)

A state of optimum capacity for effective performance of valued tasks (Parsons, 1979)

The expression of the extent to which the individual and the social body maintain in readiness the resources to meet the exigencies of the future (Dubos, 1962)

A relative state that represents the degree to which an individual can operate effectively within the circumstances of his heredity and his physical and cultural environment (McDermott, 1977).

The extent to which an individual or group is able, on the one hand, to realize aspirations and satisfy needs; and, on the other hand, to change or cope with the environment. Health is, therefore, seen as a resource of everyday life, not the objective of living; it is a positive concept emphasizing social and personal resources, as well as physical capacities (WHO, 1984)

A basic human right and essential for social and economic development (The Jakarta Declaration on Health Promotion, 1997)

These definitions suggest that health should not be thought of purely on the basis of physical fitness or the lack of identifiable disease. The concept of a holistic approach to health, where the whole person and not simply the working parts of the body are considered, has gained increasing acceptance in recent years. Many health professionals learn about their work almost exclusively in terms of diagnosis of diseases and their management and treatment. However, a person's attitudes, background, education, and culture will all contribute to their beliefs about health. There are numerous influences on health, not all of which are under the individual's control; indeed, far more are under societal or governmental control. Thus there is a limit to the effect of individual choices on health, and health professionals need to move away from the previous culture of 'victim blaming'. As pharmacists, we should therefore be aware that health involves more than pathology and therapeutics, but also embraces psychological and sociological issues, and that our view of what constitutes 'health' may differ greatly from that of the person whose health we are promoting. For example, a young person with cystic fibrosis may feel a good day to be one in which they can walk across the room unaided, or for someone with arthritis it may be to wake up without pain.

1.2   What is health promotion?

The Ottawa Charter for Health Promotion (WHO, 1986) describes health promotion as follows: 'Health promotion is the process of enabling people to increase control over, and to improve, their health'. The five Ottawa strategies for success are to: build healthy public policy; create supportive environments; strengthen community action; develop personal skills; and re-orient health services. The focus here, and it is of great importance, is that it recognizes that the individual has only limited ability to affect his health, and many more factors are under societal, governmental, and employer control. Thus a policy which focuses on individual behaviour, while not addressing the underlying factors, for example unemployment, homelessness, poor housing, and education, should be recognized for what it is—victim blaming.

The Jakarta Declaration on Health Promotion (WHO, 1997) offers a vision and focus for health promotion into the twenty first century. It recognizes that: 'health is a basic human right and essential for social and economic development' and notes that case studies from around the world provide convincing evidence that health promotion works. There is now clear evidence that comprehensive approaches to health promotion using a combination of the five Ottawa strategies are the most effective and that settings such as cities, local communities, schools, workplace, and health care facilities offer practical opportunities for the implementation of comprehensive strategies. Access to education and information is essential in achieving effective participation and the empowerment of people and communities.

As with the debate about the meaning of health, there is much philosophical debate about health promotion and there are many models, but the following have most relevance for pharmacy practice. Tannahill's model (Fig. 1.1) defines the content of health promotion rather than the practice by delineating the boundaries of health promotion, and includes negative and positive aspects of health as well as taking on a political dimension. He defines health education as 'any educational activity aimed at positively enhancing well being', prevention as 'preventive procedures' (for example immunization), and 'other preventative action' (for example self-help groups), and health protection as 'legal or fiscal controls, other regulations or policies or voluntary codes of practice aimed at the prevention of ill health or the positive enhancement of well being'. He recognizes that each of these activities can be carried out on their own or in conjunction with each other, but ignores the role of community action.

A more pragmatic solution has been adopted by Tones and Tilford (1994), who use health promotion as an umbrella term to encompass

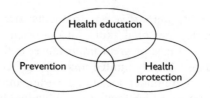

Fig. 1.1. Tannahill's model of health promotion.

all interventions that promote health, including health education. They put forward the simple formula: 'health promotion = health education × healthy public policy. Dennis and colleagues insist that 'The terms health education and health promotion are not interchangeable. Health promotion covers all aspects of those activities which seek to improve the health status of individuals and communities. It therefore includes both health education and all attempts to produce environmental and legislative change conducive to good health. Put another way, health promotion is 'concerned with making healthier choices easier choices'. (Dennis *et al.*, 1982)

The phrase 'making the healthy choice the easier choice', which goes some way to defining the philosophy of health promotion, was coined by Milio (1986). The World Health Organization also stated: 'health promotion represents a mediating strategy between people and their environments, synthesizing personal choice and social responsibility in health care to create a healthier future'. (WHO, 1986)

Beatties' structural grid (Fig. 1.2; Beattie, 1984, 1990) presents a taxonomy of health promotion that attempts to incorporate the spectrum of activities conducted. The framework identifies four discrete areas of health promotion.

1. Health persuasion: interventions directed at individuals led by professionals, e.g. encouraging a pregnant woman to stop smoking.

2. Legislative action: interventions led by professionals intended to protect individuals, e.g. lobbying MPs for a ban on tobacco advertising.

3. Personal counselling: interventions are led by individuals; the health promoter acts as a facilitator not an expert, e.g. smoking cessation clinics for individuals.

4. Community development: interventions such as those in personal counselling, seek to empower a group or a local community, e.g. smoking cessation clinics for groups.

The grid provides a means of comparing different philosophies of health promoters through analysis of the quadrant where their work originates. This was used to examine pharmacists' health promotion activities in the initial evaluation of the community pharmacy-based High Street Health promotion scheme (Todd, 1992). Todd concluded that on the whole, despite their training which explored the wider role of health promotion, the pharmacists worked from a model where the pharmacist is the expert persuading people to change.

Several approaches to health promotion have been proposed—the preventative; the radical/social change; empowerment; behaviour change; and transtheoretical. Each will be introduced briefly below.

1.2.1 The preventative approach to health promotion

Primary prevention is concerned with preventing specific diseases developing in individuals. The efforts of primary health promotion

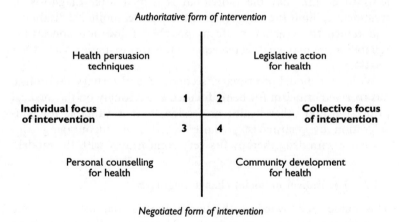

Fig. 1.2. Strategies of health promotion (Beattie, 1990).

are directed at healthy individuals, with the aim of preventing ill-health and positively improving the quality of life. Activities may include vaccination and immunization, the reduction of specific behaviours which cause disease (particularly smoking), and encouragement of general behaviour which is known to reduce health risks (for example, taking more exercise). Traditionally, health promotion and education have been identified most strongly with primary prevention.

Secondary prevention is concerned with stimulating people to respond to services for the early detection and treatment of diseases once they are established and to ensure that those treated recognize how best they can cooperate and assist with their treatment. Sometimes it may be possible to prevent the disease progressing to an irreversible stage, and secondary prevention aims to return the individual to good health. Activities might include direct patient education and screening, for example cervical and breast cancer screening programmes. When disease states occur, they do not always present with symptoms, and in these cases routine screening may be of benefit, for example the detection of congenital abnormalities in the fetus and of hypertension in adults.

Tertiary prevention ensures that patients respond effectively where the condition or disease cannot be completely cured. This aims to ensure that the individual is helped after diagnosis or treatment to limit the recurrence of the disease, minimize disability, and return to as active a life as possible. Education concerning rehabilitation may be directed equally towards ex-patients and their relatives.

While this model of primary, secondary, and tertiary prevention has received criticism for being focused too strongly on the medical profession and other health professionals, it is valuable for consideration by pharmacists, whose expertise in encouraging concordance with drug therapy fits very comfortably with the model.

1.2.2   The radical or social change approach

This model acknowledges the importance of the socio-economic environment in determining health. The goal of this model is to tackle the roots of the problems of ill-health, i e. the focus of change is society and not the individuals in it. Thus health is seen as a political issue, and policies and legislation are identified to ensure that people have access to the facilities and services they need to be healthy. The philosophy can be summed up by the phrase 'making the healthy choice the easy choice' (Milio, 1986). Examples are seat-belt legislation and no smoking policies.

1.2.3 The empowerment approach

The empowerment model (Naidoo and Wills, 1994) aims to help people to develop their concerns about health and gain the skills and confidence to act on them. Instead of acting as the expert, the health promoter acts as a facilitator, encouraging individuals to identify any concerns about their health and areas for change. This approach requires the learner to think critically about their own values and beliefs and to modify the way in which they perceive themselves.

1.2.4 The behaviour change approach

Individuals are encouraged to adopt healthy behaviour patterns, and this is seen as the key to improving health. This approach views health as the property of individuals and assumes that lifestyle changes will improve health. The Health of the Nation targets related to changing behaviour (Department of Health (DH), 1992). The last government was criticized for adopting this approach while making few of the necessary socio-economic changes.

1.2.5 The transtheoretical approach

Prochaska and DiClemente developed a model of helping people to change which incorporated a number of theoretical approaches, the transtheoretical model (TTM) (Fig. 1.3) and has been widely used. TTM is the recognition that people are in different stages of readi-ness in relation to any proposed change and that any proposed intervention should take account of this.

The stage of change that a person has reached is addressed by the health professional, who acknowledges that relapse does occur, and that people are not always ready to change 'risky' behaviours. This model has been used by the Health Education Authority (HEA) in their 'Look after your heart' and 'Helping people change' courses and for pharmacists in the Centre for Pharmacy Postgraduate Education (CPPE) workshop, *A practical approach to health promotion* (CPPE, 1996). The TTM is discussed in more detail in Chapter 4 (What makes people behave as they do, and how can behaviour be changed?).

1.3   Competencies for health promotion

Core competencies, knowledge, skills, and attitudes for those involved in health promotion have been developed (Ewles and Simnett, 1998):

1. managing, planning and evaluating;
2. communicating;
3. educating;
4. marketing and publishing;
5. facilitating;
6. influencing policy and practice.

Ewles and Simnett (1998) say it is unrealistic for all health promoters to be competent in all six areas, and that individual health promoters will also have technical specialist competencies. Pharmacists' specialist competencies include their expertise about

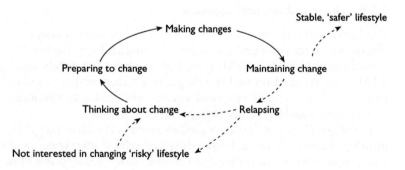

Fig. 1.3. Transthoeretical model of behaviour change (Prochaska and DiClemente, 1982, 1984).

medicines and their ability to advise on the treatment of minor ailments, to communicate informally with the public without an appointment system, to measure and advise about blood pressure, and so on. In addition, as experts, they can lobby for change.

It is, of course, important to remember that health promotion programmes can have a great impact on people's lives and that such programmes should always be evaluated to assess their benefits, disadvantages, and effectiveness. The possibility of adverse effects from any preventive measure or treatment must be set against the danger of severe illness, or even death, from the disease itself. Health advice should present a concerned person with current information about the relative risks and benefits so that any informed decision can be made.

Having considered definitions of health and the concept of health promotion, we shall now look back to the nineteenth century and describe the changes in knowledge and action in relation to health which set the scene for today's health problems and activities.

1.4 The public health movement in Victorian England (1840–1900)

The health status of most people changed very little from pre-history to the middle of the nineteenth century. Prior to the Victorian age, poverty was part of the natural order of things. In Victorian times, poverty was seen as an individual problem (the product of a deficient personal character and morality) and the poor were seen as thriftless, lazy, and undisciplined, lacking initiative and moral fibre. While the poor were to be assisted in coping with their condition of poverty, any improvement had to be achieved through their own efforts. The famous 'self-help' movement of the Victorian era was based on the premise that people were poor as a result of their own faults.

Then, as now, however, poverty was created by the economic arrangements and relationships of society which in turn determined the distribution of material resources. Power and wealth were concentrated in one sector. In a society where effective political organization was outlawed, people worked long hours in what we would now consider to be horrific conditions and for low wages.

The Poor Laws were devised with the work ethic in mind: while relief would be given to the needy, the conditions would be so harsh as to deter most—for example, by consigning them to workhouses or orphanages. The uptake of poor relief is, therefore, an inaccurate estimate of the real social conditions of those times. Of those who applied for poor relief in 1842, the reasons included insufficient wages (20 per cent), sickness (40 per cent), and old age (50 per cent). More than one reason may have been cited when claiming poor relief, hence the percentages totalling more than 100.

Against this background, crusading efforts were made to improve working-class living conditions, partly as a result of the endeavours of charismatic figures such as Edwin Chadwick who, as secretary of the Poor Law Commission in the 1830s, continued to support segregation of the needy into workhouses but at the same time advocated free elementary schooling and better sanitary standards.

Sanitary reform was essential because the fast-developing cities still relied for waste disposal and clean water on the principles which had worked in rural England, in which there was a plentiful supply of fresh water and excrement was spread on the fields. In Victorian cities, excrement flowed down open sewers and inevitably contaminated fresh water supplies. Water-borne infectious diseases such as typhoid were endemic.

There was a widespread belief that these diseases were caused by 'miasma', or bad air, and Chadwick's belief that they were water-borne was given little credence. In 1836, as a result of his efforts, death certificates began to state the cause of death and Chadwick produced 'sanitary maps' showing that most death and disease occurred in overcrowded areas and that mortality was clearly related to social class. At this time, the average life expectancy was 43 years for 'gentry' and 22 years for 'labourers'. Chadwick's *Survey of the labouring population of Great Britain* in 1842 was sufficiently comprehensive to include engineering plans showing how to build and run sewage farms and how to obtain clean water from agricultural areas. Chadwick was one of the first epidemiologists—relating diseases and their distribution to identify possible causes.

Some cities—notably Liverpool—acted immediately to improve sanitation, but most waited for the Public Health Act of 1848, which made the provisions of the Act mandatory, the stimulus being a panic engendered by an epidemic of cholera. Towns and cities were required to build drains and sewers, to pave streets, and to provide clean water. A further cholera epidemic in 1849, in which 70 000 people died, acted as an additional stimulus for the establishment of Medical Officers of Health who would in future ensure compliance with the provisions of the Act.

There was still no scientific evidence that disease was spread by unclean water, and in 1854 Chadwick was sacked for his crusading vigour, a leader in *The Times* in the same year expressing the view that 'we prefer to take our chance of cholera than to be bullied into health'. But evidence became available when a London doctor, John Snow, traced cholera deaths to a water pump in Golden Square. There were 600 deaths in that district, of which 344 occurred in 4 days, among those who drew water from this single pump. Snow traced the pipelines of various water companies and showed that one set was infected and that, when the pipes of different companies were laid side by side, those people who were served by the infected supply contracted the disease while those on the other side of the same street did not. In his report, Snow came close to anticipating Pasteur's theory of 'germs', but further time elapsed before the theory gained widespread support.

The Public Health Act of 1875 was based on the recommendations of John Simon, the Medical Officer of Health in London. This Act set standards of sewerage, controlled adulterants in food, established the quarantining of infectious diseases, and decreed the provision of infirmaries. Such legislation was justified retrospectively by the breakthrough of bacteriology in 1882, which was the beginning of medicine as a science and of disease being seen as requiring community as well as individual action. The growing power of the state made legislation easier to enforce, and its success, when enacted, further increased that power. Health became a symbol of justice and equality, replacing the concept that ill-health was an 'Act of God' on the unworthy.

The identification of causative organisms led to vaccination programmes to control infectious disease and, in the case of smallpox and diphtheria, these were significant in reducing mortality. For other diseases, the picture is neither so clear nor so obvious as one would imagine. Consider the case of tuberculosis, where it was widely believed that the advent of chemotherapy and a vaccination programme were responsible for its eradication. Figure 1.4 shows that the incidence of the disease was declining before either of those measures was introduced. Some have argued that the tuberculosis organism may have mutated or in some way become less virulent. This is possible but unlikely, since tuberculosis had been endemic in Britain for centuries. Since the condition of exposure to the disease had not changed and the slums in the early years of the nineteenth century were conducive to its spread, the strong possibility remains that improved nutrition was the factor which influenced the downward trend.

The nutritional status of the population gradually improved after the agricultural revolution. Previously there had been 'lean' years following bad harvests, and starving people are much more susceptible to disease. This is illustrated by the severe typhus epidemics, the last of which occurred in Britain in 1846–8 in the aftermath of the Irish potato famine. An improvement in diet has been postulated as a reason for the decreasing mortality of this period.

Historical analysis demonstrated that scarlet fever has shown four cycles of severity followed by remission (see Fig. 1.5), and these seem to have been largely independent of environmental conditions but due to a change in the virulence of the infective organism. From being a major killer in the early years of the twentieth century, the disease is now relatively mild, with few adverse effects. In the same way, it is thought that plague and leprosy have died out in developed countries.

Calculations show that, in the period 1838–1900, the decrease in mortality was due to the control or eradication of diseases in the following order:

Disease state	Percentage of total decrease in mortality
Tuberculosis (respiratory)	17.5%
Cholera, dysentery, and diarrhoea	10.8%
Bronchitis, pneumonia, and influenza	9.9%
Scarlet fever and diphtheria	6.2%
Typhus and typhoid	6.0%
Smallpox	1.6%

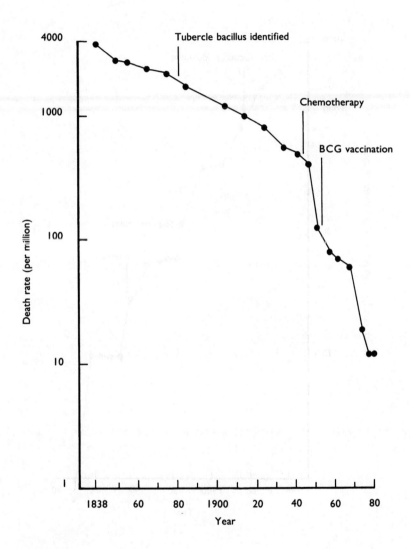

Fig. 1.4. Mean annual death rate from tuberculosis, 1838–1980. (Source: *Health, society and medicine—an introduction to community medicine,* Blackwell Scientific Publications.)

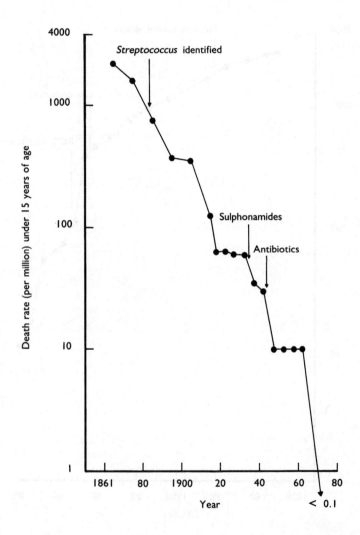

Fig. 1.5. Mean annual death rates from scarlet fever in children under 15, 1861–1980. (Source: *Health, society and medicine—an introduction to community medicine*, Blackwell Scientific Publications.)

To summarize, in the nineteenth and early twentieth century, there were few effective therapies, and much of the decline in mortality from disease was the result of preventive measures such as the Public Health Acts and vaccination programmes. While social factors such as an improvement in diet seem to have played a part, malnutrition was still a serious problem. At the turn of the 19th century, poverty, bad housing, and lack of provision for sickness and old age remained widespread.

1.5 Factors in better health 1900–47

While mortality from infectious diseases was declining by 1900, large differences remained in the rate of decline in different social groups, occupational classes, and comparative age groups. The infant mortality rate, for example, had not begun to fall by the end of the nineteenth century.

During the nineteenth century, little attention had been paid to such disparities, but two studies published at the turn of the century showed that most ill-health was suffered by the poor and that child health was the worst of all. In 1900, one study showed that only 2.5 per cent of the population claimed Poor Relief, but other surveys carried out at that time showed the reality—that one in three people were living below the poverty line.

Booth, who carried out much research into the effects of poverty, proposed a 'poverty line' below which it was impossible to provide adequate nutrition, and for the one-third of his sample who fell below it there were four main causes:

1. inadequate or irregular earnings;
2. large family size (22 per cent);
3. sickness (30 per cent);
4. old age (50 per cent).

More than one reason might apply, hence percentages totalling more than 100.

These findings were confirmed by an Inter-Departmental Committee on Physical Deterioration which was set up by the Government after one-half of the young men who volunteered for

Boer War service were rejected due to ill-health and unsatisfactory physique. The findings were published in 1904 and revealed that over one-third of children were malnourished.

Radical changes to tackle the problems of poverty and inequality were proposed by Sidney and Beatrice Webb in a minority report on the evidence submitted to the Royal Commission on the Poor Laws, which sat from 1905 to 1909. They urged the development of welfare services to attempt to remove the poor from dependence on Poor Relief. This proposal was carried into legislation which provided meals in schools (1906) and gave a pension to old people (1908). The National Insurance Act of 1911 gave some protection against sickness to working people, and the setting up of Labour Exchanges sought to alleviate unemployment. Further legislation required notification of diseases such as tuberculosis and venereal disease, and the Maternal and Child Health Act ensured the provision of maternity care, cheap infant food, health visiting, and a school health service. The fall in the infant mortality rate which occurred from the mid-eighteenth century is illustrated in Fig. 1.6.

Three factors, then, were significant in changing the health status of the nation from Victorian times to the present day:

1. public health measures, which have resulted in a clean water supply, an efficient sewage system, and a vaccination programme for the whole population;
2. fairer distribution of wealth, largely brought about by the political organization of working people;
3. a higher standard of education and knowledge of the factors which contribute to disease, which made more people aware of the ways in which they can improve their life chances.

1.6 Current inequalities in health

The Health Service Act of 1947 offered medical care to all, irrespective of economic status or geographical background. It was believed that the National Health Service would eradicate the differences in health which had existed previously. Although it seems hard to believe today, at the time of the inception of the NHS

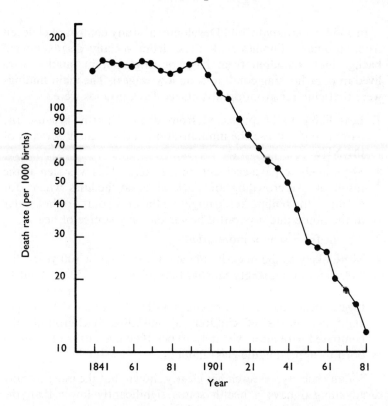

Fig. 1.6. Infant mortality in England and Wales, 1841–1981. (Source: *Health, society and medicine—an introduction to community medicine,* Blackwell Scientific Publications.)

it was widely thought that the pool of existing disease would be dealt with in a year or two. Having eradicated or cured existing disease, it was thought that the NHS would cost little to operate. In fact, the NHS has consumed ever-increasing amounts of resources and, despite the original hopes, the reality is that children of manual workers with large families, low incomes, and poor housing are still more likely to suffer ill-health and infant mortality than are those born of middle-class parents. Inequalities in health still remain, and some experts claim that the gulf between the affluent and the poor, in health terms, grows ever wider.

In 1969, a National Child Development study compared children from 'ordinary' families with those from socially disadvantaged backgrounds (children from large or single-parent families who lived in poor housing conditions on low wages). The main findings were that children from disadvantaged backgrounds were:

1. Less likely to be protected from disease, partly because the parents did not use the immunization and screening services of the NHS.

2. More likely to have accidents in the home. This was seen as the result of overcrowding and lack of basic facilities where, for example, the boiling kettle might be the only source of hot water in the house and a paraffin heater the only source of heat.

3. Absent from school more often.

4. More likely to die in early infancy. Over the past 100 years, the overall infant mortality rate has fallen from over 150 to about 15 per 1000 live births, but the relative gap between the higher and lower social classes has changed little. Approximately 30 per 1000 live births of children of unskilled backgrounds die compared with approximately 10 per 1000 live births of children born to upper-middle-class families.

For any society, research has clearly shown that the most socially disadvantaged have a health status significantly lower than the average. An awareness of this fact in situations where medical solutions are sought for what are in fact social problems helps in an assessment of how and when to offer advice on better health. When a problem is defined as an illness it becomes individual and blinds us to the more uncomfortable and harder truths of underlying social problems such as high unemployment and bad housing.

1.6.1 Inequalities in health in the 1980s and 1990s

During the 1980s, two major reports were published on the subject of inequalities in health in the UK. The first, the *Black Report*, was published in 1980 following a working group on Inequalities in Health set up in 1977 by the Secretary of State. The conclusions of the working group were that, far from inequalities in health in the UK diminishing, they were actually increasing, and that only a major and wide-ranging programme of public expenditure could set right the deep-rooted causes of those inequalities. The Government stated that the recommendations in the *Black Report* regarding public spending could not be implemented and refused to endorse them.

The Health Divide was the second major report and was published by the then Health Education Council in 1987, just before its demise. The report was written with the aim of reviewing research and statistics on inequalities in health, drawing together and summarizing the most recent evidence. Concluding that serious social inequalities in health had persisted into the 1980s, the report stated that there was strong evidence of the major impact on health of socio-economic circumstances. Using any measure of social standing, from the traditional social class categorization to more recent measures of deprivation, those at the bottom of the social scale had higher death rates and worse physical and mental health than those higher up. The numbers of stillbirths (Fig. 1.7a) and of deaths in infants aged under 1 year (Fig. 1.7b) continued to show a clear trend, with the highest rates in social classes IV and V; deaths among adults showed a similar gradient (see Fig. 1.7c).

More recently, the 1998 *Acheson Report* of the independent inquiry into inequalities in health concluded that the gap between the health chances of the richest and poorest in Britain had widened rather than narrowed.

In order to understand the evidence on social class (sometimes called occupational class) and health, the traditional categories defined by the Registrar General are as follows:

- Social class I—professional (e.g. doctor, lawyer, accountant);
- Social class II—intermediate/managerial (e.g. teacher, nurse, manager);
- Social class IIIN—skilled non-manual (e.g. typist, shop assistant);
- Social class IIIM—skilled manual (e.g. miner, bus driver, cook);
- Social class IV—semi- or partly-skilled manual (e.g., farm worker, bus conductor);
- Social class V—unskilled manual (e.g. labourer, cleaner).

The intention of this classification was to group people together who had similar living conditions and standards. The categories

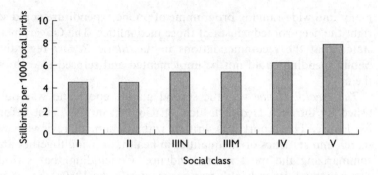

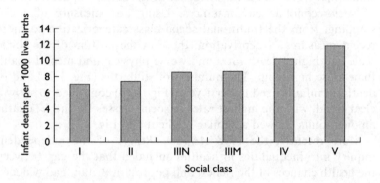

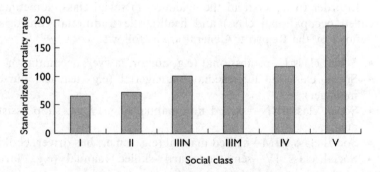

Fig. 1.7. (a) Stillbirths in England and Wales 1993–5 by social class. (b) Deaths in infants (less than 1 year) in England and Wales 1993–5 by social class. (c) Deaths in men aged 20–64 in England and Wales 1991–3 by social class. (Source: *Inequalities in health*, Office of National Statistics, 1997.)

were intended to reflect the level of wealth or poverty and the culture associated with each 'class'. Today, the classification is no longer seen as a precise measure but is still useful as a general guide for social position. Other measures of socio-economic status have since been devised which take into account, for example, car and house ownership and employment status.

Both the *Black Report* and *The Health Divide* confirmed the existence of regional differences in death rates in Great Britain. Death rates were highest in Scotland and the north and north-west of England, and lowest in the south-east of England and East Anglia. Studies had clearly shown the great inequalities in health existing between neighbouring communities and the existence of pockets of poor health corresponding to areas of social and material deprivation. The adverse influence of unemployment on health was now established through research and the national gradient of unemployment—a higher level of unemployment in the north of the country was responsible for some of the ill-health.

Socio-economic factors, while undoubtedly a major influence on health, do not explain all regional differences in morbidity and mortality. It is known that climate plays a part in health, for example ischaemic heart disease is adversely affected by cold and humidity. However, there are still large differences in morbidity and mortality from some diseases for which no explanation has yet been found, for example cancer of the stomach is 30 per cent more likely to occur in parts of Wales than in England, and the incidence of spina bifida in South Wales is among the highest in the world.

Urbanization affects disease patterns and the incidence of respiratory diseases rises in cities, partly because of increased risk of infection in crowded places and partly because of the increased pollution of the atmosphere. Occupation may affect health, but the statistics can lead to inappropriate conclusions being drawn. Experts have argued that mortality statistics for coalminers are deceptively low because workers whose health has been damaged by such work will be likely to move on to other, lighter work. Allowing for these problems, occupational health statistics can teach us a great deal about the stresses and problems of various jobs—not just the newsworthy ones of asbestos workers with damaged lungs but also the physical and 'temptation' hazards of different jobs, for example publicans have a mortality rate from cirrhosis of the liver which is eight times the national average.

In adult life, morbidity and mortality from most diseases rises with social class number, so that unskilled manual workers in social class V have the highest incidence of ill-health. There are a few exceptions to this trend, one being the incidence of malignant melanoma, a form of skin cancer. This serious and potentially fatal condition now occurs more frequently in higher social classes, and it has been postulated that this may be due to more frequent holidays in sunny climates. Death rates from breast cancer previously showed a gradient from lower to higher social classes, highest in the latter. However, more recent statistics show a more complex picture with death rates highest in social classes I/II and IV/V and lower in III. The reasons for this are not clear.

Inequality in health between groups of differing socioeconomic status is one of the most urgent issues to be addressed, and the reduction of this inequality was the first of the WHO's European targets for Health For All. The aim was that, by the year 2000, health inequalities should be reduced by 25 per cent.

1.7   Causes of disease

The endemic infectious diseases of Victorian days are now largely controlled by better living conditions, vaccination, and antibiotics. There are exceptions to this, and the increased incidence of tuberculosis in deprived populations is a cause of concern. Our environment has been rendered safer by legislation such as the Factories Acts to provide safer working conditions, firm application of the drink/driving laws, and improved living standards such as the wider availability of central heating in public housing where paraffin heaters were previously the cause of many fires. These changes have resulted in fewer accidents at work, in a commendably high standard of road safety (the UK has the lowest death rate from road accidents in the EC), and in fewer accidents in the home. This has thrown into sharp focus the diseases for which there are, as yet, no cures. For example, AIDS and some cancers (such as lung, large bowel, and breast cancer). While lung cancer death rates are falling among men, they are still increasing among women over 55. Despite many years' research and vast expenditure, cures for the major cancer killers seem little nearer. Table 1.1 shows that almost half the deaths in England and Wales are due to four causes.

1.7.1 The links between lifestyle and disease

Much research has focused on human behaviour as a cause of disease—that is to say, looking at individual lifestyles to see which behaviours may lead to ill-health. While individual behaviour undoubtedly contributes to the development of some diseases, it is accepted that government action is needed to bring about widespread change. The example of seat-belt legislation is often quoted in this context. Before the introduction of legislation on the wearing of seat-belts, large numbers of people were killed or injured each year in road accidents. Extensive advertising campaigns and exhortations to change personal behaviour were unsuccessful, and the desired behaviour change was finally achieved by legislation. In the nineteenth century, water-borne diseases were not eradicated by encouraging individuals to boil water but by state legislation.

The behaviours which are harmful to health and which we will go on to discuss now and later in this book are not solely due to a wilful disregard for health but are the result of many factors, including positive promotion by the advertising of products such as cigarettes and alcohol, of cultural and peer pressures, and of established social norms.

Smoking

Of these harmful behaviours, smoking is the greatest single cause of disease and death. Cigarettes are advertised in magazines, newspapers,

Table 1.1 Percentage of deaths in 1993 due to major diseases

Heart attack	25.3%
Stroke	10.6%
Lung cancer	5.6%
Breast cancer	4.4%

(Source: Office of National Statistics)

and at many sporting events. Each packet has a statement that smoking cigarettes may result in ill-health, introduced only after many years of pressure being exerted on tobacco companies. Smoking causes lung cancer but it is less well known by the public that it is a major cause of coronary heart disease, peptic ulcers, bronchitis, and other respiratory diseases. Of every 1000 young men who smoke cigarettes, statistics show that six will die in road accidents and 250 will die prematurely as a result of smoking. Evidence of the harmful effects of passive smoking has increased over the last decade, leading to changes such as workplace no smoking policies.

Alcohol

The cost of alcohol has decreased in real terms during the last two decades. Between 1970 and 1976, the price of beer fell by 4 per cent, wine by 14 per cent and spirits by 21 per cent compared with the Retail Price Index. Average disposable income increased by 17 per cent in real terms over the same period, thus further decreasing the true cost of alcohol. The number of licensed premises has increased, including supermarkets and off-licences, and alcohol is heavily advertised and available for purchase all day long. More recently, changes in EC legislation mean that people can, and do, buy large quantities of alcohol very cheaply and import them into the UK without tax. Alcohol intake is implicated in road accident deaths, in violence, in suicide rates, in cirrhosis of the liver, and in admission to psychiatric hospitals. While there are health benefits from moderate alcohol intake (there is evidence than an intake of one or two units a day has a protective effect against heart disease), there are significant risks from regular consumption at high levels. We do not discuss alcohol in greater depth in this book since experience has shown that pharmacy customers are unlikely to seek advice about it in the pharmacy. Pharmacists should be aware, however, of the current recommended safe limits for alcohol intake (21 units per week for women, 28 for men).

Nutrition

Our British diet now contains highly processed foods—more than ever before—and consumers often have little idea of what they are eating. Processing often removes natural fibre from foods and adds sugar, salt, and fats. Artificial flavourings and colourings make processed foods more palatable, and preservatives ensure they can be kept on the supermarket shelf for longer. Major reports published by key groups, NACNE (National Advisory Committee on Nutrition Education) in the 1980s and COMA (Committee on Medical Aspects of Food Policy) in the 1980s and 1990s, agreed that the most significant way in which our diet should change for better health was to reduce the total amount of fat and, within this, to reduce the amount of saturated fat that we eat. The traditional British diet of 'chips with everything' and large quantities of fat is an effective way to achieve a heart attack at an early age. At an individual level, people are now more aware of the importance of a healthy diet (and supermarket shelves are evidence of this, with bigger displays of fruit and vegetables and high-fibre foods). However, food purchasing also depends on access, availability, and cost. Local shops may be the only ones available to families on low incomes and without a car. The concept of 'food deserts' refers to areas where healthy food is hard to find, perhaps on council estates where local shops have closed or where shops continue to stock less healthy foods which are high in fat and sugar, and choice is limited. Similarly, fast-food outlets continue to feature high-fat foods.

Sugar

Sugar is inexpensive and therefore included in a range of foods, but the inadequate regulations on food labelling mean the manufacturer is required to state only that it is present, not its quantity. While our sugar intake is now in comparative decline, it is still a contributory factor to overweight and obesity. The prevalence of obesity is increasing. In 1994, it was estimated that 13 per cent of men and 16 per cent of women aged 16–64 were obese, around twice the rates for 1980. The prevalence of overweight for men, in 1994, was 43 per cent and was 29 per cent for women in the same age group. The addition of sugar accustoms people to its taste, and a 'sweet tooth' is established in infancy, where many proprietary baby drinks and foods have a high sugar content. For the manufacturer, the ability to add sugar means the cost of the product is reduced, sugar being cheaper than many other ingredients. All major expert reports have recommended a reduction in sugar consumption.

Salt

Salt is implicated in the incidence of hypertension and heart disease, and one-half of all the salt we eat is in processed foods, so that often we do not know when we are eating it.

Fibre

Fibre is removed from flour-based products such as bread, then salt and sugar are added. Lack of fibre is implicated as a causative factor in some cancers and bowel disease, and expert reports are in agreement that our diet should contain more fibre. The amount of wholemeal bread now consumed is rising, although the average British intake of fibre is still well below the recommended levels.

The relationship between income and nutrition

Lower income groups spend a greater percentage of their disposable income, but less in actual money, on food than do those in high-income groups. In a diet that contains excessive quantities of sugar and fats, they are likely to eat less fresh fruit, green vegetables and wholemeal bread, and more white bread and sugar. Healthy eating changes have been shown by research to have occurred more quickly and to a greater extent in people of higher socio-economic groups. The cost of many 'healthy' foods is often higher than the alternatives, for example a wholemeal loaf costs more than the standard white version.

   Differences in dietary and health choices, while undoubtedly linked to educational and cost considerations, are also likely to have cultural connotations. George Orwell noted in *The road to Wigan pier* that, if luxuries such as sweets and chocolates are the only ones which are affordable, then it is those which will be purchased. The same is true of alcohol, where price and affordability are major factors in increasing its consumption.

To add to all this, the public are often confused by frequent reports in the media on research that appears to contradict previous findings on what constitutes a healthy diet, combined with food scares which can undermine consumer confidence and contradict valid health promotion advice.

Drug misuse

The number of users of illicit drugs continues to rise. The pharmacist's contribution is through harm reduction strategies such as needle/syringe exchange, supply of prescribed substitute drugs, and supervised methadone consumption. Chapter 15 addresses the role of the pharmacist in minimizing harm from drug misuse.

Four behaviours—smoking, diet, alcohol, and lack of physical activity—are the most important areas where health promotion could have an effect, specifically on the incidence of coronary heart disease. The developments in political thinking and public policy which might focus attention on the need for these changes is discussed in the next chapter.

References

Acheson, D. (1998) *Report of the independent inquiry into Inequalities in Health*. The Stationery Office, London.

Beattie, A. (1984) Health education and the science teacher: an invitation to debate. *Education and Health* 1, 9–16.

Beattie, A. (1990) Knowledge and control in health promotion. In: Gabe, J., Calman, M. and Bury, M. *Sociology of the Health Service*. Routledge, Kegan and Paul, London.

Centre for Pharmacy Postgraduate Education (1996) *Practical Approaches to Health Promotion*. University of Manchester.

Dennis, J., Draper, P., Holland, S., Shipster, P. *et al.* (1982) Health promotion in the reorganised NHS. *Health Service Journal*, November 26th.

Department of Health (1992) *Health of the Nation*. The Stationery Office, London.

Drever, F. and Whitehead, M. (1997) *Health Inequalities*. Office for National Statistics. London.

Ewles, L. and Simnett, T. (1998) *Promoting health—A practical guide.* 4th edition. Scutari Press, London.

Health Education Authority. *Helping People Change.* HEA, London.

Milio, N. (1986) *Promoting health through public policy.* Canadian Public Health Association, Ottawa.

Naidoo, J. and Wills, J. (1994) *Health promotion: foundations for practice.* Balliere Tindall, London.

Prochaska. J. and DiClemente, C. (1982) Transtheoretical therapy— towards a more integrative model of change. *Psychotherapy: Theory, Research and Practice* 19, 276–288.

Prochaska, J. and DiClemente, C. (1984) *The Transtheoretical Approach: crossing traditional boundaries of therapy.* Dow Jones and Irwin, Homewood, Illinois.

Tannahill, A. (1985) What is health promotion? *Health Education Journal* 44, 4–5.

Todd, J. (1992) *High Street Health.* MSc dissertation. South Bank Polytechnic, London.

Tones, K. and Tilford, S. (1994) *Health Education, Effectiveness, Efficiency and Equity* (2nd edn). Chapman and Hall, London.

World Health Organization (1984) *Health promotion: a WHO discussion document, the concept and principles.* WHO Regional Office for Europe, Copenhagen.

World Health Organization (1986) The Ottawa Charter for Health Promotion.

World Health Organization (1997) The Jakarta Declaration on health promotion in the 21st century.

2 Public policy and health

In the preceding chapter, we have shown the range of factors which combine to determine individual and community health, including economic status, physical environment, occupation and education, socio-economic factors, and the provision and use of health services, as well as individual behaviour. All of these are potentially open to change through legislation and health promotion, ranging from action at community/societal level to that on an individual basis.

At the simplest level, a government policy of increasing the taxes levied on cigarettes and alcohol produces a downturn in consumption, as does banning of advertising of those products. Cigarette advertising is already banned on television, but the European agreement to ban advertising at sporting events recently has resulted in a flurry of concern and stalling actions on behalf of the British government which had massive lobbying from motor racing interests. Clearer statements on the nutritional content of food could only be helpful but, again, legislation is slow to be enacted.

However, the power of consumers continues to grow, and examples of the ways in which they have affected health outcomes include the banning of cigarette smoking on planes, in some restaurants, in cinemas, and on public transport. Using parliamentary lobbying and publicity campaigns, such groups have been very successful in raising public awareness and in achieving change.

This chapter, then, will focus on the policy changes which have brought health promotion further to the front of the government's agenda. Before doing so, it is necessary briefly to remind readers of the key drivers for change, i.e. the changed structure of the NHS, the rise of consumerist politics, and increased awareness of inequality in health and health services.

2.1   The changed NHS

During the 1980s, there were rising tensions in the NHS as new treatments became available which often had not been evaluated but were demanded by clinicians and by patients. The pressures to introduce new treatments resulted in increasingly uneven distribution of resources throughout the country, so the London teaching hospitals gained an increasing share to the detriment of other health regions, some of which had the greatest problems. This in turn resulted in increasingly bad publicity, and discussion of the problems of the NHS became commonplace on television and in newspapers. The decision was then made in the 1989 White Paper *Working for Patients* to separate the purchasing of heath care from its provision. The essential planks of this policy were to give the resource for funding the NHS to regional offices and hence to local health authorities, and to offer to general practitioners the opportunity to become fundholders. Thus local health authorities had responsibility for allocation for virtually the total resource of the NHS, initially indirectly through the regional offices of the NHS, and latterly directly. Health authorities then gave resource to fundholding general practitioners for a limited range of treatments.

While the jury is still out on the extent to which the provision of health care was altered by this radical change, most observers would agree that it did focus attention both on the cost of treatments and on the need for their evaluation. There was pressure from purchasers for providers of care to show the evidence on which new treatments were being proposed for introduction into practice, and this applied also to the rationale for introducing new medicines into widespread use. Before this separation of purchasing and provision, drug companies needed only to secure a product licence in order to guarantee that a drug, at whatever expense and however modest its improvement on previous products, would be introduced into NHS practice. So the climate within the NHS changed to one of evaluation and audit of clinical practice.While it is extremely difficult to change practices established over many years, nonetheless health authorities—guided as they are by the expertise of public health doctors, epidemiologists, statisticians, and medical and pharmaceutical advisers—are less inclined to invest in treatments where the evidence base is weak. A continuation of this philosophy is that, in the White Paper, *The NHS, a first-class service* (DH, 1998), the focus is on measuring the quality of treatment and outlining the way in which national standards will be set for services and treatments. It also describes the way in which a framework for assessing performance will be established.

In 1997, the White Paper, *The new NHS: modern, dependable* (DH, 1997), outlined the establishment of primary care groups (PCGs) to whom most NHS funds will be allocated in future. Thus decisions will be made locally to meet local health needs. Health Action Zones (HAZs) will be formed, targeting areas where greatest inequalities in health exist. Health authorities, together with their PCGs, will be required to produce a Health Improvement Programme based on local needs.

2.2   The rise of consumerism

The growth of the consumer movement has led to many changes in our society, including legislation confirming consumer rights and choices and accountability for proffered services. In the UK, patients' rights and expectations from public services were made explicit in *The Patients' Charter* (DH, 1991), which set out standards of service which patients might expect. Consumer demand has led to an explosion of information on a wide range of topics, including health; indeed, the passing of The Freedom of Information Act in the USA was consumer-driven and it is there that the consumer movement first developed. Consumer lobbying has been a powerful influence in some areas of food manufacture which involve pharmacy practice, leading, for example, to the reduction or removal of sugar from some baby foods, clearer labelling of food additives and preservatives, and their removal from many products.

To illustrate the changes that have taken place in attitudes to information provision which have impinged on pharmacy practice, it is of note that, as recently as 30 years ago, the name of the drug or medicine dispensed was not included on the dispensed medicine label. The rationale for this policy was that patients did not need to know the name of their medicine. The situation has changed so much that consumers can now access their medical records on request.

The public's demand for knowledge brings into sharp focus the dilemma of health professionals such as pharmacists and doctors, whose knowledge base previously has not been accessible to, or understood by, their clients. Knowledge has long been a source of power for professional groups, and any advance by consumers into the health knowledge base has resulted in expressed concern by health professionals that the lay person's lack of detailed understanding may lead to unfounded fears. In reality, the concern being expressed was that professional groups can regard narrowing of the gulf in knowledge between health professional and client as a threat to their professional status.

The European Community's series of directives on medicines addresses the area of patient information and requires that patient information leaflets will be issued with all medicines, giving details that include side-effects and their incidence. Thus, decisions about information giving will no longer be in the control of health professionals.

2.3   The media and health consumerism

The role of the media has been crucial in raising the level of public awareness and education about health. In particular, television programmes have accepted the consumer's right to be informed on matters of concern, including health. In some cases, the media have exposed situations where parliamentary lobbies and vested interests previously had acted to limit public availability of information. Examples of such reporting include the harmful effects of diets high in dairy products and saturated fats.

Television programmes have also provoked extensive public discussion and concern about the dangers caused by *Salmonella* in eggs, *Listeria* in cheeses, and *Escherichia coli* in meat. The transmission of bovine spongiform encephalopathy (BSE) from animals to humans has been highlighted and brought to public awareness by such programmes. The latest debate, on genetically modified products, has shown a public refusing to accept bland assurances of safety.

The development of the Internet (the World-Wide Web) has made specialist information freely available at the touch of a button for those with the resources to access the system. Political systems have discovered to their cost that they can no longer keep secret the way in which dissidents are treated within their country and, at the level of health awareness, consumers can find on the Internet all the published information on, for example, new drug treatments. Thus they come to the pharmacist or the general medical practitioner much better informed in general and specifically more knowledge-able about their disease and its treatment. As in many areas, use of the Internet currently is disproportionately high among those in higher socio-economic groups. However, the widespread use of computers in schools is likely to extend their use more widely in society.

Such articles and television programmes about the risks and benefits of drug therapy have led to a recognition among consumers that there are health choices and that an informed choice can be made about whether or not to have a particular treatment. Surgeons are now required to explain the potential benefits and risks of surgical procedures to patients. Consumers are more likely to seek further information from health professionals, such as pharmacists, who are readily accessible.

2.4   Consumers and health professionals

What consumers want from health professionals is information about their medicines and about their illnesses. Research shows that they would like health professionals to spend more time talking to them. A recent Consumers' Association study examined what patients wanted from their GP and found that over 80 per cent of respondents wished to have more information and explanation about their disease and its drug treatment. In short, they wanted their doctor to spend more time talking to them about their health. Market research involving pharmacy customers has shown that, where the pharmacist gives information and is prepared to spend time at the counter, consumers welcome this. Studies on patient information leaflets demonstrated that patients appreciated them, that they read the information contained in the leaflets, and were not put off their drug therapy by being told about common side-effects (see also Chapter 6, Concordance in medicine-taking).

Consumers' perception of pharmacists is often that they are relatively inaccessible and too busy in the dispensary. Market research shows that, whilst the pharmacist's advice is willingly given, consumers say that the consultation often had to be sought or requested rather than being volunteered by the pharmacist. Pharmacists' perceptions, on the other hand, are that they are readily accessible and available to their customers. The difference is wide.

This need for pharmacists to offer advice on health care was recognized in The Nuffield Report which was published in 1986. Its fundamental thrust for community pharmacy was that pharmacists must move towards an extended advisory role and away from a purely technical dispensing function. Within the extended role, health promotion was clearly identified by the *Nuffield Inquiry* as an area in which pharmacists should become more greatly involved, reflected in the statement that 'there is a role for pharmacists in health education in co-operation with other health professionals'.

2.5   Policy changes towards holistic health care

The White Paper *Promoting better health* was published in November 1987 (DH, 1987) and outlined future strategy and policy for primary health care. Again, health promotion was clearly identified as an important area for development in community pharmacy. *Promoting better health* contained a statement of intent to provide core funding for the provision of health education materials in community pharmacies. This promise was fulfilled in April 1989, when Kenneth Clarke, the then Secretary of State for Health, announced funding of £250 000 annually for the development of the *Health in the High Street* information scheme and other facets of health promotion in pharmacy.

Of fundamental importance for pharmacy within *Promoting better health* was the statement of intent to begin to move remuneration for community pharmacy away from the basis of dispensing prescriptions and towards the provision of other services, as Nuffield had recommended. The first such services were the provision of pharmaceutical services to residential homes and the establishment and keeping of patient medication records for elderly and confused patients. Further funding subsequently has been given to community pharmacies, via health authorities, for participation in needle exchange programmes.

In 1992, the *Health of the nation* was published (DH, 1992), which set out a strategy for health for England. It described the key health areas to be addressed and, for the first time, set targets for change. The other regions—Scotland, Wales, and Northern Ireland —had their own strategic documents for health improvement, all with a larger number of target areas than the *Health of the nation*. For the first time, health promotion was recognised by government as having a key role to play. The importance of multi-disciplinary working was highlighted, with the result that local planning groups were established with representatives from local authorities, health authorities, primary care, and other organisations.

Health of the nation targets were

1. *Coronary heart disease (CHD) and stroke.* To reduce death from CHD and stroke in people under 65 by at least 40 per cent. To reduce death from CHD in people aged 65—74 by at least 30 per cent. To reduce the death rate from stroke in people aged 65—74 by at least 40 per cent by the year 2000.

2. *Cancers.* To reduce the death rate from cancer in the population screened by at least 25 per cent. To reduce the incidence of invasive cervical cancer by at least 20 per cent. To reduce the death rate from lung cancer in the under-75s by 30 per cent in men and 15 per cent in women. To halt the yearly increase in the incidence of skin cancer by the year 2005.

3. *Mental illness.* To reduce the overall suicide rate by at least 15 per cent. To reduce the suicide rate of severely mentally ill people by 33 per cent by the year 2000.

4. *HIV/AIDS and sexual health.* To reduce the incidence of gonor-rhea by 20 per cent as an indicator of HIV/AIDS trends. To reduce by at least 50 per cent the rate of conception amongst the under-16s by the year 2000.

5. *Accidents.* To reduce the death rate for accidents among children under 15 by 33 per cent by the year 2005.

These Government health targets were based upon the population achieving lifestyle changes in four main areas:

1. *Smoking*. The aim was to reduce the prevalence of cigarette smoking to no more than 20 per cent of the population by the year 2000 in both men and women. This represents a reduction of one-third on the 1990 figure. A further aim was to reduce consumption of cigarettes by at least 40 per cent by the year 2000. More specifically, the aim was to increase the number of women who stop smoking at the start of pregnancy and to reduce the smoking prevalence of 11—15 year olds.

2. *Diet and nutrition*. The aim of the present Government policy was to reduce fat intake as follows:

   * decrease energy derived from total fat by 12 per cent
   * decrease energy derived from saturated fat by 35 per cent

   The aim was also to reduce the number of men and women aged 16—64 who are obese by at least 25 and 33 per cent, respectively, by 2005. Finally, the aim was to reduce the proportion of men drinking more than 21 units of alcohol per week and women drinking more than 14 units per week by 30 per cent by 2005 to 18 per cent of men and 7 per cent of women.

3. *Blood pressure*. The aim was to reduce mean systolic blood pressure in the adult population by at least 5 mmHg by the year 2005.

4. *HIV/AIDS*. The aim was to reduce the percentage of injecting drug misusers who report sharing injecting equipment in the previous 4 weeks from 20 per cent in 1990 to no more than 10 per cent by 1997 and no more than 5 per cent by the year 2000.

The targets have generally not been achieved due to the emphasis on the need for individuals to change their behaviour rather than for changes to be made at policy level.

2.5.1   Policy changes affecting pharmacy and primary care

For pharmacy

In August 1993, the DH announced its intentions for the longer term changes for community pharmacy. One of its policy objectives was 'to make full use of community pharmacy in primary care: by encouraging co-operation between pharmacists and GPs, providing professional advice to customers and participating in community care and health promotion programmes'. A proportion of the global sum available for pharmaceutical services has been devolved to health authorities for local purchasing of certain services.

For primary care

Primary Care: The Future (DH, 1996) lists health promotion in pharmacy as an area where innovative local practices exist and states that these innovations should be developed nationally. It proposed that pharmacists should be the first port of call for advice and over-the-counter medicines in response to common ailments. If this occurred, it said, this would increase the health promotion role. The report also said that pharmacists should be actively promoting the health of people and contributing to the local achievement of *Health of the nation* targets; and encouraging the principle of self-care and individual responsibility for health. 'People are unwilling to take responsibility for their own health. Educate people to use the pharmacist as professional adviser and pharmacists to become more than shopkeepers'. The report acknowledged that there should be changes in remuneration away from perverse incentives, and towards increased working with the primary care team, and that there was a major constraint due to the pharmacist having to be on the premises constantly for supervision. The report also called for improvements in pharmacy premises, to create a more professional atmosphere and to provide private counselling areas or space for more health promotion material.

For the population

The White Paper *Our Healthier Nation* (DH, 1999) mentioned community pharmacists as part of the whole NHS which will take responsibility for the success of the health strategy and will work together to achieve it. It focused on improving the health of the population as a whole by increasing the length of people's lives and the number of years people spend free from illness. It seeks to improve the health of the worst off in society and to narrow the health gap. Four major target areas are included: coronary heart disease and stroke; cancer; mental health; and accidents (see Chapter 3). The paper calls upon local purchasers to develop Health Improvement Plans (HImPs) and to change services to deliver appropriate heath care effectively. Health care providers, including pharmacists, are to be held responsible for their contribution in making people healthier. It is noted that all health professionals approach health from a different perspective and with different expertise and that all have a role to play.

The new NHS: modern, dependable

The White Paper, *The new NHS: modern, dependable* (DH, 1997) emphasized the need for the NHS to work locally to reduce inequalities in health and to improve health. It highlighted the need for health promotion and introduced the idea of Health Improvement Programmes which will be joint plans to improve health and health care locally. The paper acknowledged that 'most people look to their family doctor or local pharmacist for advice on health matters'. Quality is important, and national indicators of quality will be developed. Primary care groups will be set up and these will involve pharmacists in the planning and provision of services. Health Action Zones will be formed, targeting areas where greatest inequalities in health exist. Pharmacies in these areas will have the opportunity to develop as part of 'healthy living centres'.

Thus the policy statements and direction of funding have, over the past 20 years, moved from a strictly medical model of health and into recognition that a range of factors affects the way in which people make decisions about their health and their life style. The ways in which pharmacists can help in decision making will be described in Chapter 4.

References

Department of Health (1987) *Promoting Better Health*. HMSO, London.
Department of Health (1989) *Working for Patients*. HMSO, London.
Department of Health (1991) *The Patients' Charter*. HMSO, London.
Department of Health (1992) *Health of the Nation*. HMSO, London.
Department of Health (1997) *The new NHS: modern, dependable*. The Stationery Office, London.
Department of Health (1998) *Our Healthier Nation*. The Stationery Office, London.
Department of Health (1998) *The NHS, a first class service*. The Stationery Office, London.

3 Major health challenges facing the 21st century

If they are to be effective in the role of health promoters, pharmacists need to be aware of the major diseases, the extent to which they can be prevented, and the importance of environmental and social as well as biomedical influences. Another key issue is, for each disease area, the extent to which pharmacists have a unique contribution to make, and can become involved through collaborative working with nurses, doctors, social care workers, and others. Such joint working will essential. This chapter will set out the major health challenges in the context of long-term government and health service priorities, and ways in which pharmacists can play their part.

In England and Wales, government priorities for reducing ill-health in the next decade are those set out in *Our Healthier Nation* (there are equivalent policy documents for Scotland and Northern Ireland):

- Heart disease and stroke
- Cancers
- Mental health
- Accidents

Other health priorities

As well as the four national priority areas, the intention is that Health Improvement Programmes will also include a small number of local health priorities. *Our Healthier Nation* listed asthma/respiratory diseases; teenage pregnancy; infant mortality; back pain/rheumatism/arthritis; environment; diabetes; oral health; and vulnerable groups (for example different minority ethnic groups, homeless people). Pharmacists can make a contribution to many of these areas, and can work with other local agencies to include these.

Our Healthier Nation recognizes that good or poor health is the result of a combination of social, environmental, and biomedical factors. If the death rates of people doing manual jobs were the same as those doing non-manual jobs, 42 000 fewer people aged between 16 and 74 would die each year in England and Wales. Health Action Zones (HAZs) and Healthy Living Centres (HLCs) will be set up, initially in areas of social deprivation, and all stakeholders will have the opportunity to work together within these to improve health. The four national target areas in *Our Healthier Nation* will form the major components of local Health Improvement Programmes, and pharmacists will have opportunities to contribute. The targets were selected, states *Our Healthier Nation*, 'because they are significant causes of premature death and poor health, there are marked inequalities in who suffers from them, there is much that can be done to prevent them or treat them or to treat them more effectively, and they are real causes of public concern'.

Another feature of government policy on health is that National Service Frameworks (NSFs) are being developed for the delivery of NHS services, the first two being Coronary Heart Disease and Mental Health. These frameworks use current evidence to define appropriate interventions and services, and will set out standards for service provision across both primary and secondary care.

Our Healthier Nation seeks to reduce mortality figures by introducing more effective preventive measures. Almost 90 000 people die before their 65th birthday each year in England and Wales. Cancer is the cause of death of almost 32 000 of these, and heart disease, stroke, and related illnesses are responsible for a further 25 000.

Targets have been set by the government for the year 2010 to enable progress to be measured.

- *Heart disease and stroke*—to reduce the death rate from heart disease and stroke and related illnesses amongst people under 65 by at least a further third from the 25 000 in 1996.
- *Cancer*—to reduce the death rate from cancer among the under-65s by at least a further fifth from the 32 000 in 1996.
- *Mental health*—to reduce the death rate from suicide and undetermined injury by at least a further sixth from the 1996 baseline.

- *Accidents*—to reduce the rate of accidents resulting in a hospital visit or GP consultation by at least a fifth from the 1996 baseline.

Approaches to reducing ill-health and death from chronic diseases have, until quite recently, been based on evidence about risk factors. The theory, therefore, was that by influencing risk factors, health would be improved. The main method of achieving this was through encouraging individuals to change their behaviour, particularly diet, smoking, and exercise. Recent years have seen growing evidence that a person's chances of disease later in life are 'programmed' before and at birth. There is, therefore, a growing emphasis on antenatal and early life care and their importance in influencing health risks.

3.1   Heart disease and stroke

3.1.1   Epidemiology

The UK continues to have one of the highest rates of death from circulatory diseases in Europe (third highest after Ireland and Finland) (see Fig. 3.1).

Death rates from heart disease and stroke in both men and women have been falling in recent years. However heart disease and stroke are still responsible for some 18 000 deaths in men (one-third of all deaths in men) and 7000 deaths in women (one-fifth of all deaths in women) aged under 65 in England and Wales. Coronary heart disease is the result of atherosclerosis, where deposits of cholesterol and other lipids on the artery walls leads to a narrowing of the vessels, gradually restricting blood flow.

Contrary to public perception, coronary heart disease is more prevalent in manual than in professional working groups. The old image of the stressed executive, vulnerable to a heart attack, which drew attention to the disease in the 1960s, still persists. The extent of inequalities is shown by the fact that men of working age in the lowest (unskilled) social class are 50% more likely to die of heart disease than are men in the total population. Differences in smoking rates are a key factor, since those in higher socio-economic groups are much less likely to smoke. However, smoking status

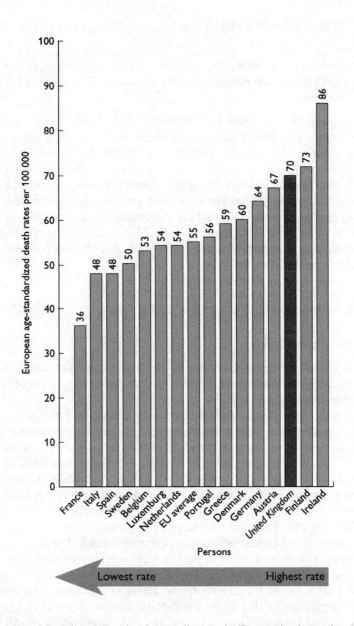

Fig. 3.1 Mortality from circulatory diseases in Europe in the under 65s. (Source: WHO Health for All statistical database; *Our Healthier Nation*, 1998). Note: Data for 1995 except Austria 1996; Denmark and France 1994; Ireland, Italy and Spain 1993; Belgium 1992.

alone cannot explain the level of difference in mortality, and nor can the other well-known risk factors for heart disease. The Whitehall study is one of the most famous epidemiological studies of heart disease. Following a large group of male civil servants, it looked at death and illness from heart disease according to individual risk factors and employment grades. Over a 10-year period, men in the lowest grade had three times the number of deaths from coronary heart disease as those in the highest. The researchers have suggested that their findings can be explained, to an extent, in terms of the level of control that an individual has over his daily work. People working in the lower grades, it is argued, have less control, and this in some way contributes to the development of heart disease.

Research has provided some indications as to which other factors might be playing a part and these are outlined below.

3.1.2   Risk factors

1. *Age, gender, family history, ethnicity, socio-economic status, poverty*—risk increases with increasing age. Men are more likely to die from heart disease and at a younger age than are women. Those with a family history of heart disease are themselves at higher risk. These factors, although recognizable, are of course not modifiable. Poverty and deprivation result in a higher risk of heart disease which cannot totally be explained by individuals' behaviour.

2. *Smoking*—this is the single most important modifiable risk factor. Since one in four of all deaths from coronary heart disease have been estimated to be due to smoking, stopping smoking is the action which can have the largest effect in reducing risk. Those who have had a heart attack can reduce future risk by half by stopping smoking. Smoking itself has a direct causal effect on stroke and is an independent risk factor. All smokers who quit will benefit through reduced risk of stroke.

3. *Alcohol*—high alcohol consumption is associated with raised blood pressure and thus increased risk. However, low to moderate intake has a protective effect against heart disease.

4. *Blood cholesterol*—it is the ratio of lipids which is important. Raised low-density lipoprotein (LDL) increases risk, as does lowered high-density lipoprotein (HDL). Blood lipid levels are subject to genetic determination to some extent, but are also closely related to intake of saturated fats. Reducing total dietary fat as well as saturated fat is a key health message in reducing obesity.

5. *Blood pressure*—hypertension is a risk factor for both heart disease and stroke

6. *Overweight*—being overweight or obese puts additional strain on the heart and increases risk.

7. *Diet*—eating a diet high in fat (particularly saturated fat) increases an individual's risk of heart disease. Diets high in salt and sugar contribute to heart disease through increased blood pressure and obesity, respectively.

8. *Physical activity*—lack of exercise has long been recognized as a risk factor. Studies have shown that as a society, we take too little exercise. This is partly due to the shift in types of employment, such that jobs involving physical activity are less common. There are other explanations, for example widespread car ownership and the reduction in the amount of time which schoolchildren spend in P.E. classes.

3.1.3   Other factors

Stress is widely perceived as a major risk factor for coronary heart disease. This perception probably has its origins in early research on personality type and heart disease (the Type A/Type B personality theory). The exact role of stress in the causation of heart disease is unquantified.

Ther is some evidence that growth retardation during fetal development leads to higher risk of heart disease. The exact mechanism whereby this occurs is as yet unknown. Other epidemiological research indicates that infancy and even pre-infancy conditions can have a lifelong effect on health chances. Poor nutrition in pregnancy appears to increase the child's risk of having heart disease in later life. The exact mechanisms by which this happens are not yet fully understood. Such research is filling out the picture of causative factors in heart disease.

3.1.4 Interventions

Primary prevention seeks to prevent specific diseases developing in individuals and includes encouragment to reduce specific behaviours (smoking, for example) and increase others (exercise). Secondary prevention aims to prevent diagnosed heart disease from progressing and is implemented after a person has heart disease (for example following a heart attack or the diagnosis of angina). Thus the main interventions the pharmacist can implement are based on encouraging lifestyle changes and on the use of medicines.

Large-scale studies have attempted to change modifiable risk factors through lifestyle change in the general population, the thinking being that if blood pressure and blood cholesterol levels could be reduced across populations, deaths from heart disease would be reduced. However, these studies met with limited success and were costly to implement in whole populations. Evidence therefore suggests that for lifestyle changes, health promotion activity is most effective when targeted at high risk individuals, and that tackling one risk factor at a time is most likely to produce an effect. Government interventions involving legislation and education policies to produce societal change are effective and powerful and have a potential effect far greater than the encouragement of individuals to change. That is not to say that work at individual level is not worthwhile, rather that both are needed.

Medicines are now commonly used as interventions in both primary and secondary prevention. The key ones are:

Primary prevention
  Nicotine replacement therapy
  Antihypertensives, e.g. thiazide diuretics, beta-blockers, ACE inhibitors
  Lipid-lowering agents, e.g. statins (also used in secondary prevention)
Secondary prevention
  Antiplatelet agents, e.g. aspirin, dipyridamole
  Beta-blockers and ACE inhibitors after myocardial infarction

3.1.5 The pharmacist's role

Pharmacists can contribute to reducing ill-health due to heart disease by:

- supporting concordance in medicine-taking (see Chapter 6)
- encouraging and advising on smoking cessation (see Chapter 7)
- offering information and advice about healthy eating (see Chapter 8)
- encouraging regular exercise (see Chapter 9)
- learning cardiopulmonary resuscitation skills
- targeting advice for those patients receiving treatment for heart problems and at risk of heart disease and stroke (using patient medication records to find patients taking relevant medicines)

3.2 Cancers

3.2.1 Epidemiology

Over 245 000 new cases of cancer were registered in the UK in 1995 and these figures exclude non-melanoma skin cancers (an estimated 40 000 new cases). Four types of cancer (lung, breast, colorectal and prostate) account for half of all new cases. Cancer is the second leading cause of death, responsible for a quarter of deaths (130 000, of whom 32 000 are aged under 65). On current rates of incidence, one in three people will develop cancer at some time in their lives. About a quarter of cancer deaths are from lung cancer and a further quarter from colorectal, breast and prostate cancer.

The degree to which cancers are preventable has been the cause of debate, but it is thought that 80 per cent are potentially avoidable. Cancer is largely a disease of old age, and almost three-quarters of new cases occur in people aged over 60. Pharmacists need to be alert for signs and symptoms which might indicate the early stages of cancer and refer accordingly. The extent of variation by social class is shown by the fact that, overall, the death rate from cancer in unskilled workers is twice that in professionals. For some cancers, the differential is even greater, for example lung cancer, where the rate is four times, and stomach cancer where it is three times higher in unskilled workers than in professionals. Some of the commoner cancers are usually too advanced for curative treatment by the time they are diagnosed. The main way to improve survival is by strategies aimed at prevention and early detection. Lifestyle changes are a key preventive measure, and earlier diagnosis and treatment can increase survival chances. Pharmacists can advise on the former and encourage the latter by early referral of suspicious symptoms, and promotion of screening services to increase uptake.

3.2.2   Risk factors

Smoking and diet are the two major modifiable risk factors for cancer, and in terms of health education priorities these are far more significant than other risks. One in three cancer deaths is associated with smoking. Eating a diet high in fat increases the risk of cancer.

3.2.3   Interventions

Prevention and early diagnosis are targeted at breast, cervical, lung, colorectal, and malignant melanoma of the skin. Screening programmes for breast and cervical cancer enable early detection and have been shown to save lives. Public education on the early signs of cancer can play an important role. Countries such as North America and Australia have been very pro-active in this respect, with major programmes on prostate, bowel, and skin cancer.

3.2.4   The pharmacist's role

Pharmacists can contribute in two main ways—helping to speed up the detection of cancer, and giving advice on prevention:

- early referral of patients with symptoms which are suggestive of early signs of cancer (see sections on individual cancers below)
- encouraging and advising on smoking cessation (see Chapter 7)
- offering information and advice about healthy eating (see Chapter 8)

The European 10-point cancer code summarizes the key health education points for cancer prevention and is a useful reference point for giving advice.

The European 10-point cancer code

1. Stop smoking
2. Stay within safe alcohol limits
3. Avoid being overweight
4. Take care in the sun
5. Observe health and safety regulations at work
6. Cut down on fatty foods
7. Eat plenty of fresh fruit and vegetables and other foods containing fibre
8. See your doctor if there is any unexplained change in your normal health which lasts longer than 2 weeks (e.g. a change in bowel habit)
9. and 10. (For women) Have a regular cervical smear test and examine your breasts each month

3.2.5 Lung cancer

This is the leading cause of cancer deaths and almost entirely preventable—over 90 per cent of all lung cancer mortality is attributable to smoking. Survival from lung cancer is low. Lung cancer is the cause of the highest number of cancer deaths in men (22 000 in 1996). Among men, the rate of lung cancer has been falling, but the opposite is true in women, because of changes in smoking rates. Levels of smoking among schoolchildren in the UK show that more teenage girls are beginning to smoke than are boys.

Stopping people starting to smoke is the key aspect of prevention. Health education activities in schools and other community locations are an important component. Banning tobacco advertising is, however, the most important action in stopping new smokers. For existing smokers, promoting and supporting smoking cessation is the major intervention. Pharmacists are in a unique position since they control access to most nicotine replacement therapy.

Community pharmacists are frequently asked to advise on treatments for cough. Any persistent unexplained cough (particularly if associated with blood in the sputum and any degree of breathing difficulty) needs to be referred. Any cough which starts in a smoker and becomes chronic is a sign for referral. Other symptoms such as blood in the sputum and unexplained weight loss are further indicators of serious pathology. The incidence of lung cancer rises steeply with increasing age, and pharmacists should be aware of the need for referral of chronic cough in older people. Unexpected and unexplained weight loss in someone middle-aged or older is a strong indication of serious disease, especially cancer.

3.2.6   Bowel (colorectal) cancer

Colorectal cancer is the second most common cause of deaths from cancer in the UK. Each year there are over 30 000 new cases and 20 000 deaths. Half of all patients with colorectal cancer present late, so the prognosis is poor.

Prompt referral of prolonged changes in bowel habit (3 weeks plus)— if detected in the early stages, the prognosis is promising. Pharmacists need to be alert for signs and symptoms which suggest the possibility of bowel cancer. Bowel cancer is relatively rare in the under-50s so early signs should be considered in the 50 plus age group. A prolonged (more than 3 weeks) and unexplained change in bowel habit is an indication for referral. Rectal bleeding and unexplained weight loss are further indicators of serious pathology. Risk factors for bowel cancer include a family history of this cancer, or of polyps in the bowel (polyposis), or a history of inflammatory bowel disease (Crohn's disease or ulcerative colitis).

Public health education about early signs—pharmacists can stock leaflets on bowel cancer and its early symptoms and signs.

Health education on diet—many studies have shown an association between bowel cancer and a diet that is high in fat (particularly red meat consumption), and low in fibre. Eating a diet that is lower in fat protects against both cancer and heart disease.

The evidence on fibre has become clearer in recent years. Insoluble fibre increases bulk in the intestine, in turn leading to food passing more quickly through the gut. Food takes longer to travel through the intestines with a diet low in fibre, and this is thought to expose the wall of the gut to carcinogenic substances in foods and to allow the conversion of some substances into more harmful forms.

Large epidemiological studies have indicated that lower levels of specific vitamins (A, C and E) and minerals (selenium) may be linked to increased rates of certain cancers, but the evidence is complex and not definitive. The advice to increase intake of foods containing these substances would be reasonable, but routine use of dietary supplements cannot be recommended on the basis of current evidence. Selenium is toxic if ingested in amounts greater than the recommended dose.

3.2.7 Breast cancer

Over 25 000 new cases of breast cancer are diagnosed in women each year and some 15,000 women die annually from this cancer. The UK has seen a fall in mortality from breast cancer in recent years. This is thought to be due to both earlier detection and more effective treatment. Breast cancer is rare in men, with around 170 new cases and 100 deaths annually. While women are probably unlikely to consult their pharmacist rather than their GP about breast symptoms, an important role for pharmacists is stocking leaflets on breast self-examination. Evidence shows that regular self-examination is the most effective way to identify breast lumps.

Encouragement to take up mammography—mammography programmes have been shown to reduce breast cancer mortality by almost a third. Routine screening by mammography is now offered to all women aged between 50 and 64 and repeated every 3 years. The screening technique is less effective in women aged under 50, and further research is investigating the reasons why.

Currently women from more advantaged backgrounds are more likely to participate than those from deprived backgrounds. The reasons for this are to do with education and understanding of the potential benefits of screening and also access to services (car ownership is higher in the higher socio-economic groups). Pharmacists can work with other local services to publicize screening programmes and their benefits.

Recommending a diet low in fat—there is some evidence that a diet high in fat increases the risk of breast cancer, by promoting cancer rather than initiating it. Excessive fat intake, resulting in obesity, has been linked with breast cancer. This effect had been shown in post-menopausal women, and more recent evidence suggests that high fat intake and obesity in the early childhood years (up to age 10) increases the risk of breast cancer. However, this is an area where the evidence is not definitive and the findings of studies have been conflicting in some cases.

Information about medicines and breast cancer risk—pharmacists have an important role in information-giving about possible increased risk. Many women are concerned about the increased risk of breast cancer from hormone replacement therapy (HRT). In fact this risk is small, and the benefits and risks can be put into context (see Chapter 12). Pharmacists are important 'translators and interpreters' of evidence for the public, since they are the most accessible health professionals. They are therefore in a position to be able to increase the patient's involvement in decisions about treatment where information requires clarification and explanation.

3.2.8   Cervical cancer

Some 2000 women die of cervical cancer each year in the UK. Research evidence indicates that cervical cancer may be caused by a sexually transmitted agent, possibly a genital wart virus. Known risks are early age of first intercourse and multiple sexual partners. A woman's risk is also increased by the number of sexual contacts her male partner has had. Recent trends have been an increase in deaths in younger women (aged between 25 and 34) and a decrease in deaths in women aged 45 and over. Barrier methods of contraception can reduce the risk of cervical cancer, and it is thought that trends in mortality may be related to changing patterns of contraceptive use (particularly use of the oral contraceptive pill as the sole contraceptive method). With the advent of HIV/AIDS and the protective effect of condoms, the use of barrier methods has increased and this may have an effect on cervical cancer rates.

Survival rates are very good for women whose cancer is detected and treated early. Screening through the 'smear' test is intended to reduce the incidence of and mortality from cervical cancer by detecting and treating pre-cancerous conditions. Women aged 20–64 should have a smear test every 3 years. More than 80 per cent of invasive disease is found in women aged over 35, many of whom have never been screened. Highly publicized failures in local screening services, where tests were classified inaccurately, led to deaths from cervical cancer and are (understandably) likely to have resulted in a loss of confidence among women.

Encouragement to take up cervical screening—women from deprived backgrounds are less likely to attend for smear tests, and pharmacies in deprived areas have a particularly important role in promoting women's participation in screening. This can be done by working with other health agencies and community groups to publicize screening through leaflets and posters.

Smoking cessation—smoking appears to increase susceptibility to cervical cancer.

3.2.9   Malignant melanoma and other skin cancers

Pharmacists have a unique role to play here since many skin cancers are preventable through appropriate protection against the effects of the sun. This is important for exposure to the sun at home, and on summer and winter sun holidays, including ski-ing. Sunscreens are a key part of the strategy to prevent these cancers (See Chapter 14 for specific advice on sunscreens).

The commoner types of skin cancer (basal cell carcinomas) occur mainly in the elderly and account for some 10 per cent of all cancers in this country. These cancers are seldom fatal, since they very rarely metastasize and can be cured. Basal cell carcinoma (also known as rodent ulcers) occur mainly on the head and neck. The less common squamous cell carcinomas may also present as ulcers.

Malignant melanoma is a far rarer skin cancer, accounting for about 1 per cent of all skin cancers. However, this cancer is also one of the most deadly, causing deaths in 1997 of 326 men and 271 women. The chances of cure are very good if treatment can be carried out at an early stage of the melanoma's development, before it has begun to spread (metastasize). Outlook also depends on the thickness of the cancer—there is very good survival for those with 'thin' tumours. Early detection is thus crucial, as is public education about when to seek medical advice about suspicious moles or other lesions.

Excessive exposure to the sun, particularly over short periods of time, and bad sunburn, in childhood as well as in adulthood, is known to be associated with an increased risk of malignant melanoma. Thus, as the number of people taking holidays in sunny countries has increased, so has the incidence of melanoma. Between 1974 and 1984, the number of new cases increased by over half, from 1735 to 2626 and since then to the 1999 estimate of 3860 (2160 in women and 1700 in men). Melanoma is one of the few cancers to have a significant impact on young adults, although it is extremely rare in childhood. One in five of those who develop melanoma are aged under 40 (compared with less than 5 percent of all cancers). Those most at risk are fair-skinned, fair or red-haired, with light-coloured eyes, who never tan or burn before they tan. Also at risk are those with a large number of ordinary moles (over 60 in young people, over 50 in older people). Unusual moles which change shape (large, irregular, and multi-coloured) are another risk factor. A further factor is a family history of melanoma, or having previously had a melanoma.

There are several types of malignant melanoma, the commonest of which is superficial spreading melanoma. This may start from a mole or freckle and is often on the lower leg in women and on the back in men. Nodular melanomas account for about one-quarter of all melanomas and are commoner in men, often occurring on the trunk. They grow relatively rapidly and may bleed at a fairly early stage. A third type of melanoma is slow-growing and often occurs in people aged over 60, frequently on the cheek. A fourth type can arise in and around the nail bed, especially on the big toe.

Early referral of suspicious lesions—in around one-third of cases, the melanoma develops from a pre-existing mole:

Major skin signs for referral to the doctor:

1. Is an existing mole getting larger or a new one growing? After puberty, moles do not usually grow.

2. Does it have a ragged outline? Ordinary moles are smooth and have a regular shape.

3. Does it have a mixture of different shades of brown and black? Ordinary moles may be quite dark brown or black but are all one shade.

Any of these may also be present in a melanoma:

4. Is it bigger than the blunt end of a pencil? Most normal moles are smaller than this.

5. Is the mole inflamed or does it have a reddish edge? An ordinary one is not inflamed.

6. Is it bleeding, oozing, or crusting? Ordinary moles do not do this.

7. Is there a change in sensation, such as a mild itch? An ordinary mole is not usually itchy or painful.

(From the Cancer Research Campaign, 'Be a mole watcher')

3.3   Mental health

3.3.1   Epidemiology

Mental health problems are widespread. The 1996 Health Survey for England showed that 20 per cent of women and 14 per cent of men may have had a mental illness. The figures are not precise since many patients may not present to formal health services because of the perceived stigma of poor mental health, or because they do not recognize that they are ill. Under-diagnosis of depression, for example, has been identified as a major problem, and the Royal College of Psychiatrists has been running its 'Defeat Depression' campaign for several years. The evidence suggests a trend over the last three decades for increasing numbers of children and young people to suffer mental health problems, particularly those from disadvantaged social backgrounds. Further evidence of inequalities in the incidence of poor mental health is demonstrated by the figures for suicides, where men of working age who are unskilled workers are more than twice as likely to commit suicide than are those in the overall population.

3.3.2   Interventions

Medicines are a key intervention in mental health problems, although there are complex issues relating to concordance and compliance (See Chapter 6 for a general discussion of these issues). Pharmacists learn about the biochemical changes underlying conditions such as depression and schizophrenia and see treatment with medicines as a logical way to set right the imbalance. However, the patients who experience the diagnostic process and resulting treatment seee things from a very different perspective. Trying to see the patient's point of view is an important precursor to any intervention aimed at increasing compliance. Pharmacists have an important role in encouraging patients and their partners, relatives and carers to discuss the treatment. Giving information and support to patients' parents, partners and carers is a key role.

One of the key issues involves the 'medicalization' of mental health problems, and some argue that the use of medicines does not address underlying problems. Some patients feel that being prescribed a medicine is not an appropriate response to their perception of the problem. Patients may feel that the medicine makes them feel different (tiredness, suppression of emotions) and may perceive this as being worse than the original problem itself. They may be concerned that the medicine is addictive and that they will become dependent on it, even where there is unlikely to be any physical or psychological dependence. Such concerns may not be overtly expressed. The older drugs used to treat depression and schizophrenia tend to have more unpleasant side-effects such that patients may decide not to take them.

The use of 'talking' therapies has increased in recent years, and patients generally have welcomed this move. Cognitive therapy has been shown to be effective in the treatment of depression, and family therapy is of demonstrated effectiveness in schizophrenia. The term 'Counselling therapy' is often used in a non-specific way, often not well defined, and this is probably the reason why evidence for the effectiveness of counselling is not definitive.

The use of exercise and relaxation techniques to reduce stress are suggested in *Our Healthier Nation*. The health challenges of trying to reduce the use of alcohol and smoking to combat stress are well recognized.

3.3.3   The pharmacist's role

- Liaising with mental health outreach services, especially community mental health nurses

- Targeting advice to new prescriptions; monitor progress and asking patients about side-effects
- Using PMRs to find patients taking relevant medicines and target support
- Providing information about self-help groups
- Supporting concordance in medicine-taking (see Chapter 6)
- Encouraging exercise and activities to reduce stress (see Chapter 9)

3.4   Accidents

3.4.1   Epidemiology

More deaths in children and young people are due to accidents than to any other cause. Home-related accidents are the most common cause of childrens' deaths above the age of 1 year. In 1996 there were 3640 deaths in England and Wales as a result of an accident in the home. Some 1.5 million hospital treatments and 1.2 million GP consultations are due to home accidents.

3.4.2   Risk factors

The commonest home factors which feature in accidental deaths are shown in Table 3.1.

Table 3.1   Most frequent causes of accidental death in the home in 1994

Cause	Estimated number of deaths
Stairs/steps in or out	524
Fire (uncontrolled)	288
Food/drink	210
Aspirin/analgesics	197
Other medicines	182
Alcohol	135
Bed	72
Cigarettes	56
Chair	54
Fire (controlled)	50
Carbon monoxide	40

(Source: DTT Home Accident Surveillance System Annual Report 1997)

Children from the poorest backgrounds are five times more likely to die as a result of an accident than are those from better off families. The reasons for this are complex and inter-related, but we will give some examples here. The risk of fires is increased in homes where the family cannot afford the cost of installation of central heating and where gas heaters, for example, are used. Smoking-related fires are also more likely, since smoking rates are higher among more deprived groups. Families living in poverty are less likely to know about and be able to afford safety equipment such as smoke detectors, stair gates, and so on.

At the other end of the age spectrum, accidents, especially falls, are a major cause of disability and death in older people.

The possible role of prescribed and non-prescribed medicines in road traffic accidents has been the subject of recent research. There is an important educational need in ensuring that people understand the potential effects of reduced reaction times and even slight drowsiness.

3.4.3   Interventions

A quarter of the one million people who are injured in, or die from, falls in the home every year are aged over 65. Pharmacists can consider which medicines might increase the chances of a fall and monitor their effects.

Osteoporosis is a major source of problems following falls in elderly people, and the treatment of high-risk groups to prevent osteoporosis is a key intervention. Hormone replacement therapy and other preventive treatments are crucial, hence the importance of the pharmacist's input in ensuring their use.

3.4.4   The pharmacist's role

Some 400 people die each year in reported accidents resulting from the intake of medicines. The use of child-resistant containers (CRCs) has reduced the incidence of medicines poisoning in children. The Royal Pharmaceutical Society of Great Britain (RPSGB) policy on CRCs is that pharmacists should offer ordinary closures where a person has problems opening a CRC. Pharmacists can remind older people about the importance of secure storage of medicines, especially where grandchildren are likely to be visiting.

Pharmacists can also help by monitoring treatment and giving advice to support prevention of accidents:

- Having an appropriate and practical policy on the use of CRCs and taking part in DUMP campaigns
- Offering information about treatments for osteoporosis and monitoring their use (see Chapters 6 and 12)
- Offering advice about smoking cessation (see Chapter 7)
- Long-term preventive advice about healthy eating, and obtaining sufficient calcium and vitamin D (see Chapter 8)
- Encouraging regular exercise in younger people to build and maintain bone strength (see Chapter 9)
- Informing local businesses about first aid requirements and stocking an appropriate range of kits and equipment
- In the role of community advocate, encouraging general measures such as the use of smoke alarms and electric socket covers
- Supervising methadone consumption to reduce quantities in the home (Chapter 15).

4 How can behaviour be changed?

Health professionals often struggle to understand what makes people persist with behaviours that are harmful to health. There is a commonly but erroneously held view that simply giving information will change behaviour. Research shows this not to be the case. In intervening to promote health, the aim is not to somehow manipulate people to follow our own agenda. Rather, it is to provide information and respond to queries in a non-judgemental way such that people can make their own, informed choices about behaviour. For health professionals, this means accepting that sometimes people will choose not to follow healthier options. Information and advice can be tailored to individuals' needs by learning from the findings of psychology research. Advising, educating, and persuading people to adopt healthier lifestyles are the core skills required of pharmacists in health promotion. In this chapter, we will explore the reasons why people pursue unhealthy behaviours, present a model for behaviour change that pharmacists can use in their everyday practice, and provide an introduction to the necessary communication skills.

4.1   Why do people pursue unhealthy lifestyles?

It is often assumed that people smoke, eat unhealthy foods, do not exercise, and do not take their medicines because of a lack of information. Yet surveys show that the health risks, for example of smoking, are well known throughout the population. Why then, when large numbers of people understand that smoking and eating fatty foods can lead to coronary heart disease, do many people continue to smoke and to consume foods which are not the most healthy? If pharmacists are to offer advice that has any chance of being accepted, it is essential to have an understanding of some of the reasons underlying continued behaviours which pose a risk to health.

In fact, people undertake their own risk–benefit analyses. Smoking might be a way of maintaining desired weight, or of coping with social disadvantage because it is seen as 'helping to unwind'. Educational, social, and cultural background all play a major part in determining a person's response to ill-health and attitude towards maintaining good health. Underlying attitudes determine the extent to which particular issues are addressed or avoided. These attitudes and beliefs may or may not be openly acknowledged or expressed by pharmacy customers. They may not even be recognized as such by the individuals who hold them.

Attitudes to food, for example, are formed early in life, and research has shown that it is easier to influence the diet of younger than older children. Food preferences are strongly influenced by the social and environmental context in which food is offered to children. Pairing nutritious foods with additional parental attention resulted in these foods becoming more attractive to children in one study; illustrating the inter-linking of foods and emotional relationships. The formation of attitudes and behaviour towards food in the early years helps to explain the findings from numerous studies showing that achieving long-term changes in eating patterns is difficult.

Cigarette smoking, too, is a behaviour with social and emotional overtones. People who start to smoke as a member of a peer group may come to associate smoking with friendliness, a feeling of 'belonging', and enjoyment. These underlying attitudes are targeted in campaigns which emphasize the antisocial nature and dirtiness of smoking.

4.2   The influence of health beliefs

Attitudes and beliefs about health are developed by the social and political context in which they arise, and by a process of social learning. The ability of the pharmacist to influence people's behaviour is affected by the health beliefs of both the individual and the pharmacist. Positive attitudes towards the prevention of ill-health are fundamental, and health professionals need to maintain a non-judgemental approach if their advice is to be accepted.

Several sociological and psychological models have been put forward to extend our understanding and explain people's behaviour in relation to health. The 'Health Belief Model' and the Theory of Reasoned Action are two of the most widely known and suggest that actions taken to maintain health, or respond to ill-health, are related to the perceived seriousness and risks involved and the perceived benefits of taking the particular course of action or treatment being offered. Numerous factors influence health behaviour, and one key skill for the pharmacist might be defined as 'persuading' in order to encourage people to consider and possibly change behaviour.

4.3 Understanding of risk

Research has shown that people have widely varying concepts not only of what constitutes health but also of the nature of health risks. One study showed that, of 100 men under the age of 60 who had had a heart attack, 85 smoked but only one in three believed that smoking had anything to do with their heart attack. Many of these men had seen or heard information which suggested that smoking and heart disease were linked, but their health belief was that this was not the case. Instead, many believed that stress was the most important factor in the development of their condition. More recently, in a survey where members of the public were asked about possible health risks of passive smoking, while the majority knew that lung cancer was a possible risk, only half knew that heart disease was also a risk.

The communication of risk to the public has been the subject of much research in recent years. In particular, producing user-friendly information about the size of a health risk and the extent to which that risk might be reduced has been a major challenge. Recent attempts have used visual approaches and tried to relate the risk to concepts with everyday familiarity. One example is the use of the idea of streets, towns, counties, and countries to put risk in perspective. For example, a 1 in 100 risk might be related to a street, a 1 in 100 000 with a town, a 1 in 1 000 000 with a county, and so on. Information could then be related to the local area.

Even more difficult to get across are the concepts of relative and absolute risk, where research shows, for example, that the behaviour of prescribers is influenced by the way in which data on risk reduction is presented to them, for example in published clinical trials. Reduction in relative risk has a more powerful effect than reduction in absolute risk. It is only by developing meaningful information of this type for both the public and for health professionals that people will be able to make informed decisions about behaviour.

4.4   Risk–benefit assessments

Essentially, people make health choices by making their own estimate of the likely physical and emotional consequences of their actions, in effect a risk–benefit assessment. This estimate may be favourable or unfavourable, and behaviour is maintained or altered depending on the person's subjective assessment of the likely outcomes. The outcome of the assessment is sometimes referred to as 'decisional balance', or relative weighting of the pros and cons of making a change, and it is shifts in decisional balance that ultimately will lead to changes in behaviour.

There are two aspects in individuals' risk–benefit assessments: beliefs and evaluation. Taking smoking as an example, a smoker may know and accept that they will have an increased risk of dying prematurely from lung cancer or heart disease. On the other hand, the immediate value of smoking as a coping strategy in a difficult life is one factor which will affect the decision to stop, because the person's belief about smoking may be that they will be unable to cope with everyday life without it. The long-term benefits of quitting smoking, i.e. living longer, may not be attractive to someone whose life is unhappy and poor. The smoker may also believe that the health damage has been done and that there is therefore no benefit to be gained by stopping.

Thus, clients do not always follow patterns of behaviour and lifestyle which are the most conducive to good health, even when information is available to them. There are two major issues in health promotion activity for the pharmacist: the educational aspect, which presents information, and the pharmacist's interpersonal skills in communicating health messages and persuading people to modify their behaviour.

4.5   Models of behaviour change

In recent years the 'Transtheoretical Model' (TTM), more commonly known as the 'Stages of Change' model, has become widely used. Developed by Prochaska and DiClemente in the 1970s and 1980s, the model draws on theories from psychotherapy to explain variations in people's response to advice about changing behaviour and to set out a framework for tailoring advice to individuals. The model presents five stages:

Stage	Behaviour	Implications for pharmacist intervention
Pre-contemplation	The individual is content with current behaviour and has no intention of changing; is not considering change	Listen and respond to questions. Attempts to persuade unlikely to be successful.
Contemplation	The person is thinking about the possibility of changing, but has made no plans to change.	Listen and respond to questions. Provide information.
Preparation	The decision has been made to change and the person is getting ready to make the change	Help in planning and goal-setting.
Action	The change is implemented	Encourage return to pharmacy to discuss progress. Supportive approach.
Maintenance	The person works to prevent relapse to the previous behaviour.	Continue supportive approach. Encourage discussion of possible problems that might lead to relapse. Give positive feedback.

The principle of 'Stages of Change' is that for intervention to be successful, it must match the stage the person is currently at. The sequence of stages is not linear and is best viewed as a cycle. The person can, at any stage, loop back to an earlier stage and go through the cycle again (see Fig. 1.3, p. 8). The goal of pharmacists' intervention is to move the individual forward through the cycle at a pace which responds to their own needs and choices. The challenge for the health professional is to identify an individual's current stage, i.e. their 'readiness to change'. There is no point in trying to offer information to someone at the pre-contemplation stage, nor in attempting to persuade them that they need to change. Pharmacists' time is limited and is better targeted at the stages where it is more likely to be effective. The pharmacy environment can be used to promote the availability of information and advice such that when people reach the contemplation stage they view the pharmacy as a valid source of help.

The model has been tested most widely in the treatment of addiction and dependence in studies, for example, of smoking cessation and alcohol dependence.

There have been relatively few trials using 'Stages of Change' in the short intervention times which are likely to occur in community pharmacy and primary care. However, a recent community pharmacy-based randomized controlled trial of smoking cessation showed a significantly higher rate of successful quitting among people in the intervention group, where 'Stages of Change' was used. Given that community pharmacists often know their regular customers and patients well, it might be expected that such existing knowledge and relationships might shorten the time required for interventions.

4.6   Counselling and advice-giving

Before going on to consider the interpersonal skills needed for pharmacists to communicate effectively with clients and with other health workers, we will first discuss the different types of inter-actions between pharmacist and client—counselling, advice-giving, and instruction. Counselling and advice-giving are sometimes considered to be synonymous, and pharmacists often use the term 'patient counselling'. In fact the two terms describe approaches which are fundamentally different, and it is important to understand their differentiating features.

4.6.1 Counselling

Couselling has been defined as 'the means by which one person helps another to clarify their life situation and to decide upon further lines of action', and its aim is 'to give the client an opportunity to explore, discover, and clarify ways of living more resourcefully and towards greater well-being'. Most pharmacists would agree that this is not the activity in which they are generally involved. Counselling seeks to enable or empower the patient or client to decide on a particular course of action and see it through. The key point is that the counsellor is helping the client to make their own decision, even if that decision is different from the one the counsellor thinks they should make.

Key skills in counselling include listening, empathy, and negotiation. To demonstrate the principles of counselling and the negotiation of a course of action which is acceptable to the client, consider the following list which describes changes that may take place after counselling. These personal changes are based on observation and evaluation of clients who have gone through the counselling process.

- The person comes to see himself differently
- They accept themselves and their feelings more fully
- They become more confident and self-directing
- They become more flexible, less rigid, in their perceptions
- They behave in a more mature fashion
- They become more accepting of others
- They change their basic personality characteristics in constructive ways

(Adapted from Rogers, 1967)

Counselling takes place in a variety of situations, many of which are relevant to health, including drug misuse and alcohol misuse, and pregnancy termination (the latter including genetic counselling where genetic defects may be or have been identified). HIV testing is now commonplace and, while home testing kits have been suggested, the need for counselling has meant that the test is not available without it.

We suggest that generally, counselling is not what takes place in community pharmacies and that pharmacists are involved primarily in the giving of information and advice which suggests or directs the course of action that the client or patient should take. While pharmacists may sometimes use the skills of counselling, they are largely concerned with giving information to clients and trying to ensure that this information is understood.

4.6.2   Advice-giving

Advice-giving describes the transfer of information and advice about recommended actions from the pharmacist to an individual patient or customer. Ideally, advice-giving should be a two-way interactive process, where the person is invited to respond and to seek further information should they need it. Advice-giving in relation to prescribed medicines may be generated in two types of situation. The pharmacist may offer advice or the patient may request it. Here, explaining skills are vital, such that the patient understands the information that they have been given. In responding to symptoms, the pharmacist's advice relates to a request from the person, and questioning skills are also important in determining the possible cause of the problem and formulating appropriate advice. Opportunistic health promotion advice can be offered in relation to prescription medicines and in response to symptoms. Here, the person has not asked the pharmacist directly for such advice but the opportunity arises through the symptom or medicine being discussed. Research suggests that pharmacists tend not to offer unsolicited advice, perhaps because they are concerned that it may not be welcomed. However, providing the advice is introduced in a neutral and non-judgemental way, the pharmacist can then assess the person's initial response and decide whether to continue further on that occasion. For example, in questioning someone who has sought advice about treatment for a cough, the pharmacist may find that the person is a heavy smoker and could ask a simple question such as 'have you ever thought of stopping?' Depending on the response, the pharmacist can draw on the 'Stages of Change' model to decide what to do next. If the person's response indicates they are at the contemplation stage, the pharmacist might then offer written information on smoking cessation to be taken away and read. Another example would be in discussing treatment a for baby's nappy rash, offering advice on nappy changing and skin care to prevent recurrence.

4.6.3 Instruction

In the third and last form of interaction, instruction, the input is the pharmacist telling the person what to do, in effect directing them as to what action to take. Examples here would be the pharmacist reinforcing the instructions on a medicine label by verbally repeating key items, or explaining how to use an inhaler in asthma treatment. Good instruction should be a two-way process, with the pharmacist inviting feedback from the individual.

4.7 Which communication skills are required?

The elements of good communication have been described extensively by other authors. Here we will briefly comment on the essential features of interpersonal communication and their relevance to pharmacy practice and to health promotion. Written communication in the form of leaflets is a mainstay of the provision of information about health and is a valuable means of reinforcing verbal advice, so this is also considered. A list of further reading on communication can be found at the end of this chapter.

Communication should be a two-way process between pharmacist and patient or customer. One of the myths about communication is that 'good communicators are born, not made'. This is not true. An awareness of the rudiments of the skills needed, preferably combined with communication skills training and followed by reflection on the pharmacist's own practice, can produce substantial improvements in an individual's ability to communicate. Undergraduate pharmacy programmes now incorporate communication skills training and development.

4.7.1 Listening skills

'Being a good listener' is as much a skill as a natural state. The verbal and non-verbal features which make a speaker recognize that they are being listened to can be learned and practised by the pharmacist. Non-verbal signs, including establishing and maintaining eye contact, smiling, nodding, and the use of posture (in leaning towards the patient), all signify that the listener is paying attention. Conversely, avoiding eye contact, a bored or inattentive expression or behaviours, a posture which leans away from the patient, doing more than one thing at once, and interrupting all suggest that the listener is not paying attention. Verbal signs can indicate that careful listening is going on, and these include occasional comments which do not interrupt the flow of conversation from the speaker. Thus, nodding of the head can be supplemented by brief verbal contributions such as 'Yes', or 'Mmm'. Questions and comments can also be used to show interest, create empathy, and demonstrate listening, examples being 'Did he?', 'Really?', and exclamations such as 'Oh no!', 'How awful/wonderful/embarrassing', and so on.

Listening without interrupting is one of the hallmarks of a good listener. Sometimes it is difficult not to interrupt what a patient is saying, for example if a factually incorrect statement is made, or something with which the pharmacist strongly disagrees. Interrupting is sometimes a way of controlling or time-limiting a discussion, and may be done subconsciously, especially in a busy pharmacy where the pharmacist is aware that there are other demands on their time. While it may be considered a counsel of perfection to say 'never interrupt', the practical implication is that the pharmacist needs to be aware of the effect of interrupting.

In practice, everyone has experienced the feeling that they are not being listened to, and in this respect it is invariably the non-verbal rather than verbal signs which are the most telling. When verbal and non-verbal messages conflict, for example if the listener says 'How interesting' while at the same time looking at their watch, or picking up a document and reading it, the speaker will believe the non-verbal message.

4.7.2 Questioning

There are basically two types of questions—open or closed. To illustrate the difference, if a pharmacist was going to advise a client about stopping smoking, an open question would be 'Tell me about your smoking', and the equivalent closed questions might be a series such as 'How many do you smoke a day?', 'When do you smoke?', 'Where do you smoke?', 'Why do you want to stop?', and so on.

Open questions are generally known to produce lengthier answers and can thus be more time-consuming. Such questions also generate information in an unstructured and unpredictable way. Listening skills are of key importance in sifting the emerging items of information. The advantage of open questions is that they allow patients to put forward the information that is important to them rather than responding to someone else's agenda, and that they encourage the expression of feelings, attitudes, and emotions. In the context of health promotion, open questions can produce information which helps the pharmacist to better understand the person's goals and motives. Typical opening phrases might be: 'Can you tell me about ... ?', 'Can you describe ... ?'

One approach which takes into account the limitations of time in most pharmacist–client interactions is the 'funnel' technique. Here the pharmacist begins with one or two open questions and then gradually narrows the focus of the consultation by asking a series of less open questions. In reply to a question such as 'What's the best thing for a headache', the pharmacist might first ask 'Can you tell me about the headache?' or 'What's the headache like?', thus inviting the person to give their views and thoughts. The subsequent line of questioning will be based on the information received, summarizing and checking, allowing the focus of questioning to be developed. The focus of later questions will thus narrow, for example 'So you've been having headaches for about a week and it hurts all around your head. Have you noticed any other symptoms before or during the headache?', 'Can you think of anything that might be causing the headaches?' Then, 'So you haven't had any other problems, just the headaches, and you've been very busy at work recently', and so on.

4.7.3 Explaining skills

Our research has shown that pharmacists often give people many items of information in an unstructured way during explaining and advice-giving. Studies have shown that most people will only remember three or four items of information from a verbal explanation, so this needs to be taken into account in planning explanations. Supplementing verbal information with written information is valuable, and the pharmacist can use a leaflet to highlight the key points. A useful structure for explanations is:

1. introduction (what is going to be explained and why)
2. information, then
3. summary.

The pharmacist begins by introducing the explanation which is to be given and briefly showing its relevance and importance. For example, 'I'm going to tell you how to increase the fibre in your diet. This will help to stop your constipation coming back. This leaflet shows you the three easiest ways to increase fibre in the diet ...'. And then, 'So after you've started eating the food with more fibre, you need to drink more fluids—that's really important'. Simply by saying 'this is very important' the pharmacist can flag up the value of the information to be given. The use of numbering sequences can also be helpful. For example, in the above exchange, the pharmacist identifies that there are three pieces of information which are important, and this can be emphasized further by the use of 'firstly, secondly and thirdly' before each section. Repetition of the most important points is another means of improving recall. Finally, a demonstration, for example of how to find information about fibre on food labels, can be effective.

Feedback should be asked for by the pharmacist at the end of any explanation to check that the person has understood. To continue with the example on dietary fibre, the pharmacist might obtain feedback by asking the person to relate the information to their own diet and give examples of how they might change it. Research in pharmacies shows that pharmacists, like doctors, rarely check whether the information they have given has been understood, and this is an area for improvement.

4.7.4 Language and jargon

There are many ways in which language can influence the communication process; some are listed below:

• Accent
• Regional dialect

- Regional phrases and terms
- Language barrier/English not first language
- Limit of vocabulary
- Use of jargon

The vocabulary and language used by the pharmacist are a major influence on the customer's understanding. During their training, each health professional learns the technical language or jargon associated with their professional group. It then becomes all too easy to speak in terms which the lay person cannot understand. The vocabulary range of many members of the public is limited and, generally speaking, the higher the educational level, the wider the vocabulary. Pharmacists need to bear this in mind constantly so that they stick to simple terms and avoid jargon and technical terms wherever possible. Examples overheard by the authors in pharmacies include:

1. A young hospital pharmacist had just dispensed a prescription for a young child for sustained release capsules:

   Pharmacist: So it's one capsule morning and night
   Mother: She's only 7, she'll never be able to swallow these. Can I tip the powder into some jam?
   Pharmacist: Well the thing is, they're sustained release
   Mother (ignoring the pharmacist's statement): But can I tip them out onto some jam so she can swallow it?

2. Experienced community pharmacist responding to a request for information about an over-the-counter medicine:

   Customer: What about those Ibuprofen tablets then, how do they work?
   Pharmacist: It's a non-steroidal anti-inflammatory
   Customer (bewildered): Oh, I see

Such examples are common. Pharmacists are not trying to 'blind people with science' but they sometimes forget that customers do not have the same vocabulary. Where the use of a technical term is unavoidable, the term should be introduced and then explained.

The pharmacist may speak a different language from their customers. Our research in pharmacies in inner-city Birmingham with a high proportion of Asian customers showed a significant number of pharmacies where neither the pharmacist nor their staff could speak the main language of their clients. Where the pharmacist does not speak the language, recruiting members of staff who do is a priority action.

Health professionals often believe, incorrectly, that people from minority ethnic groups are illiterate. Such thinking is based on the situation that was prominent many years ago, with first-generation immigrants to this country. As the number of first-generation immigrants declines and more family members learn to speak and read English, the situation is changing. Checking with the local Health Promotion Unit is valuable to confirm which languages are spoken locally and whether any leaflets in these languages are available.

4.7.5 Influencing/persuading skills

The list below sets out the ways in which pharmacists can use their own image, the pharmacy environment, and effective interpersonal skills to become more effective influencers:

Guidelines for becoming a 'persuasive pharmacist':

1. Think about your personal appearance—do you dress and look like a professional? First impressions are crucial in developing positive expectations among the public.

2. Think about the appearance of your pharmacy—does it have the appearance and atmosphere of a professional environment? How might you change it?

3. Raise your status and credibility by providing high-quality services and information to individuals and to local groups and causes. Take up opportunities to demonstrate your expertise, for example by acting as a source of advice to local newspapers and other media, and by giving talks at local schools and organizations

4. When talking to clients and patients, try to find something in their background that is similar to yours—people are more persuasive if they are perceived as having something in common with the people they are trying to persuade.

5. Use simple language and offer as much information as the person wants.

6. When your clients and patients present ideas that do not coincide with yours, give them additional ideas and viewpoints to think about. When a list of opposing views is presented to someone, the last one tends to be the most persuasive and remembered.

7. Strong statements tend to be less effective than a series of milder ones.

8. At the beginning of your persuasive argument, state clearly what behaviour change is needed.

9. Involve the individual in formulating their action plan rather than trying to enforce your own plan. Use the 'Stages of Change' model. A negotiated series of actions is more likely to be followed.

10. When presenting a series of facts or emotional appeals, also present a summary and conclusion, rather than leaving the person to draw their own conclusion.

11. Remember that, over time, even the most persuasive behaviour and attitude changes tend to diminish. Invite the person to return and discuss progress and reinforce changed behaviours to prolong their effects. Praise effort, progress, and achievement, however small.

12. Find a positive value, attitude, or behaviour held by the person and express positive feelings about it. Develop this positive aspect and use it in your persuasive approach.

(Adapted from *Communication skills in pharmacy practice*, Tindall *et al.*, 1989)

4.7.6 Using written information

Given that patient recall from verbal information is low, written information can be an effective method of reinforcement and supplementation. Provision of written information as patient information leaflets with prescribed medicines became compulsory at the end of 1998. Pharmacy computer systems can also generate information leaflets, and general practitioner software increasingly can do so. The readability and understandability of these leaflets will be variable. The information they contain may not be consistent.

So, although the use of leaflets is fast becoming universal, it is important to remember that, even when designed and distributed with the best of intentions, the leaflet may not be read, understood, or remembered.

Research and experience have shown that the kind of written information used is critical to its success. The type and complexity of language used are major factors—the average reading age of the British population is 6–7 years. One patient information expert suggested that the language used should resemble that in the most commonly read daily tabloids, such as *The Sun*, since that was the kind of written information many members of the public would be most familiar with.

The typeface used must be sufficiently large to allow it to be read by those with poor or failing eyesight. Layout and the use of illustrations have also been found to influence whether a leaflet is read. There is no point in having leaflets containing excellent information if they will not be read by the intended audience.

One way in which pharmacists can increase the likelihood of the leaflet being read is to incorporate it into the explanation, highlighting the relevant items. This is one way of reducing the time spent giving verbal information.

The pharmacist needs to be familiar with the content of leaflets stocked in the pharmacy. When the supply of 'Pharmacy Healthcare Scheme' or health authority sponsored leaflets arrives, pharmacists and assistants should spend a few minutes reading each leaflet and thinking about how it might be used in explanations.

4.7.7 Maximizing understanding and memory

We have outlined simple ways in which pharmacists can increase patients' and customers' memory and understanding of the health promotion advice they are given. A summary of effective information-giving is given below:

- Speak slowly
- Avoid jargon
- Use short words and sentences—simplification
- Increase recall—minimize the number of facts given
  —select the most important
  —stress the importance

—specific rather than general
—repetition
* Written back-up—readability
—physical format—typesize, colour, quality of print, and paper
—link with verbal information
Encourage feedback—check understanding
(Adapted from *Communicating with patients*, Ley, 1988)

Further reading

Ewles, L. and Simnett, I. (1998) *Promoting Health: A Practical Guide* (4th edn). John Wiley & Sons, Chichester.

Hargie, O. (ed.) (1986) *A Handbook of Communication Skills*. Croom Helm, Beckenham, Kent.

Hargie, O., Saunders, C. and Dickson, D. (1987) *Social Skills in Interpersonal Communication*. Croom Helm, Beckenham, Kent.

Katz, J. and Peberdy, A. (eds) (1997) *Promoting Health: Knowledge and Practice*. The Open University/Macmillan Press, Milton Keynes.

Ley, P. (1988) *Communicating with Patients*. Croom Helm, Beckenham, Kent.

Tindall, W., Beardsley, R. S. and Kimberlin, C. L. (1989) *Communication Skills in Pharmacy Practice*. Lea and Febiger, Baltimore.

5 Health promotion in pharmacy practice and primary care

The promotion of health and the prevention of disease are now seen as a priority for the health service. The pharmacist's role too needs to develop to reflect this shift in emphasis away from simply treating those who are ill. Within primary care, Health Improvement Programmes (HImPs) and Health Action Zones (HAZs) will be key to the development of activities to promote health during the next decade. Community pharmacies increasingly are recognized as an important delivery point for health promotion as they are visited by the healthy as well as the sick. In this chapter, we will trace the historical background to the development of the pharmacist's role in health promotion, discuss the nature of that role, consider the emerging infrastructure, and look to future developments.

5.1 Historical development of the pharmacist's role in health promotion

The first mention of health education in the *Pharmaceutical Journal* was in 1964 when a pharmacy-based dental health campaign in the West of Scotland was reported. During the 1960s and 1970s, the health education role was put forward as a 'good idea' for pharmacy, but few initiatives actually began. During the 1980s, a number of significant health promotion projects involving pharmacies were underway, including smoking cessation, blood pressure measurement, healthy eating, prevention of heart disease, and safe storage and use of medicines. In a farsighted development, the Family Planning Association (now known as fpa) started to work with community pharmacies through the Royal Pharmaceutical Society of Great Britain (RPSGB) from 1981, distributing a range of family planning leaflets through pharmacies. The Pharmacy

Healthcare Scheme (PHS), which still exists today, grew from this collaboration. In the meantime, some pharmacists were becoming involved in health screening, and training in health promotion for community pharmacists was being provided in the West Midlands and Northern Ireland. The mid-1980s also saw the first undergraduate health promotion programme at Aston University's School of Pharmacy. In 1986, the first UK-wide pharmacy-based health promotion initiative was launched, 'Healthcare in the High Street' (now known as the Pharmacy Healthcare Scheme or PHS). The late 1980s saw the establishment of the first community pharmacy-based needle and syringe exchange schemes. The first studies to report on cholesterol testing services in pharmacies were also published at around this time.

The next major landmark was the Barnet 'High Street Health Scheme' (HSHS). Launched in 1991, this was the first health authority-sponsored scheme. The Barnet scheme acted as a stimulus to other health authorities to involve and train pharmacists in health promotion. While these developments were positive, the constraints to the further development of health promotion in community pharmacy were confirmed as those that were first highlighted in the 1960s: namely lack of time, money, space, and training.

5.1.1 The Pharmacy Health Care Scheme (PHS)

The 'Healthcare in the High Street' campaign was launched in 1986 by RPSGB, NPA, the FPA, Health Education Authority (HEA), and the Health Education Board for Scotland. Later, Boots the Chemist, Health Promotion Wales, and the Pharmaceutical Society for Northern Ireland became involved in the scheme. The scheme provided pharmacists with a free leaflet stand and a monthly supply of health education leaflets on one topic, thus enabling national coordination.

The initial aims were: to provide free leaflets from pharmacies to members of the public on all major health care concerns; to provide a non-threatening, easily available, non-medical source of professional information on major health care issues; and to extend the health care role of the pharmacist in ways which would not replace but complement existing health care service provision in a cost-effective and beneficial way.

In 1989, the Government allocated £250 000 to support the scheme and continues to allocate money on an annual basis. In 1992, a limited company was formed to administer and develop the scheme, which was then renamed the Pharmacy Health Care Scheme.

Evaluations of the PHS in England and Wales during the 1980s showed that leaflets were available in the majority (over 90 per cent) of community pharmacies, although not always on open display, and that the leaflet stand was used in just over half of pharmacies. A Scottish survey in 1987 showed that 68 per cent of customers reacted to PHS leaflets in a positive way, while the remainder were indifferent. Those organizations whose leaflets were featured in the PHS reported a strong response from the public. A leaflet on Alzheimer's disease resulted in 1200 inquiries to the Alzheimer's Disease Society within 3 weeks. The British Heart Foundation reported 14 000 requests for further information in the 3 months following a leaflet on coronary heart disease.

In 1993, the first national evaluation of the PHS was commissioned. Pharmacists' views about their role in health promotion were examined along with an investigation of the number and range of leaflets available, the means by which the leaflets were distributed to the public, and the usual extent of uptake. Views were also collected on the appropriateness and the content of the leaflets and about whether the scheme met the pharmacists' requirements and whether they believed it to be useful to the public. Ninety two per cent of pharmacists said they had heard of the scheme. One in six of more recently registered pharmacists had not heard of it, and half of this group felt that they were not informed enough about it. Most pharmacists claimed that leaflets were displayed or left somewhere where customers could help themselves; hardly any said they did not display leaflets at all. The majority said that 'all' or 'most' of the leaflets were, 'just picked up' by people and only a few were taken on the pharmacist's recommendation, suggesting that the pharmacists' role in the scheme was largely the passive enabling of leaflet distribution rather than a more active input. Four out of five pharmacists believed the leaflets to be useful to the public; two out of five said it helped them to promote health to the public.

Since 1994, pharmacists have been remunerated through the professional allowance (part of the NHS contract for community pharmaceutical services) for displaying such health promotion leaflets, posters, and publications as the health authority may approve. The pharmacy is required to display up to eight leaflets at any one time, although pharmacists may stock more if they wish to do so. The incorporation of this requirement into the criteria for the professional allowance ensured its wide application in practice as well as providing a mechanism for greater liaison between the Local Pharmaceutical Committee and the health authority.

5.1.2 Education and training

Health promotion only reached widespread exposure in pharmacy education and training in the 1990s. The Secretary and Registrar of the Royal Pharmaceutical Society asked for Regional Health Authorities to provide training in health promotion as early as 1970, but provision was variable. In 1990, the Department of Health distributed the first module of a distance learning course for pharmacists, *Health Screening for Health Promotion*, to all community pharmacists in England. The increasing importance placed on health promotion was highlighted by the RPSGB's Council call for the inclusion of health promotion in the core undergraduate pharmacy curriculum in 1990. This was followed in 1991 by a Council of Europe statement that it was essential for pharmacists to have education on health education and communication skills, to increase their confidence and participation. Health promotion is now included in all undergraduate and many postgraduate courses, as well as in continuing education programmes.

5.1.3 Evidence base for the pharmacist's role in health promotion

There is increasing evidence on the quality, acceptability, and effectiveness of the role of pharmacists in health promotion. The randomized controlled trials conducted in Scotland and Northern Ireland of pharmacists' intervention in smoking cessation have shown clear outcomes. The Aberdeen researchers have published data which have shown that pharmacists trained to make brief interventions using the 'Stages of Change' model gave effective advice on smoking cessation. Customers who were counselled by these pharmacists were significantly more likely to have stopped smoking after 9 months when compared with customers advised by pharmacists in the control group.

Evaluation of pharmacy health promotion initiatives has tended to be limited and not sufficiently rigorous. Within health promotion, there is a continuing debate on appropriate methodologies for evaluation, with the recognition that randomized controlled trials cannot answer all of the important questions. The result of this debate is that pluralistic approaches are now considered to be the way forward. Maguire and colleagues at Queen's University Belfast showed that it was feasible for pharmacists to be involved in effective health promotion campaigns, health screening, and smoking cessation services while running a busy dispensing pharmacy. One health authority, Somerset, attempted to quantify pharmacists' health promotion activity as part of a health promotion scheme. The study design compared six 'test' pharmacies (receipt of health promotion training) with four 'usual care' (volunteers); balanced by five 'usual care' (selected by the health authority). Pharmacists used a simple log to record their health promotion activity over 8 months in smoking cessation, pregnancy, sun and skin protection, blood pressure monitoring, peak flow measurement, and infestations. Of the 2103 consultations recorded, the test group recorded higher numbers. The test group also held the highest number of consultations lasting more than 6 minutes and the lowest lasting 1 minute or less. A major limitation was that self-recording of consultations could measure the quantity but not any effect the training may have had on the quality of advice that was given. The validity and accuracy of self-reporting are, of course, questionable without any means of confirming the data.

The Barnet scheme (HSHS) was evaluated in a number of ways including in-depth interviews, customer surveys, audit, and covert participant research. The main findings in relation to consumers were that regular pharmacy customers were the highest users of the service and that, in general, consumers did not perceive giving health advice as part of the pharmacist's role. The participating pharmacists reported changes in their attitudes and practice, and these were also observed during the covert research. Participants reported that they were more likely to be involved in health promotion and to make interventions that were informal and opportunistic, linked to sale or supply of medicines. They also reported being more involved in advice-giving on diet, smoking cessation, and asthma, spending less time dispensing medicines and more time talking to and advising patients and using health promotion leaflets appropriately. Prior to training, time and lack of training were the largest barriers perceived by both Barnet HSHS pharmacists and controls. After the scheme had been established, lack of remuneration was the largest barrier to involvement in health promotion perceived by the HSHS pharmacists.

Other studies have concluded that the main constraints to pharmacist involvement in health promotion are lack of time, space, finance, and training, and a perceived conflict between the professional and commercial roles of the pharmacist.

In the evaluation of another health authority-based scheme in Wiltshire, participants reported that health promotion training had led to changes in knowledge, and perceived changes in attitude and practice. The participants' change in attitude, towards a more holistic view of health, was seen by the researchers as a positive benefit of training. Changes in practice were evident despite recognized constraints. Several recommendations were made of relevance to future health promotion training schemes: training should be ongoing; joint working with other health care professionals is needed to fully achieve training objectives; the role of the pharmacist should be promoted; and this currently unremunerated role should be recognized by the health authority for its potential contribution towards the health care of the population, and receive appropriate funding.

5.1.4 Consumers' attitudes to health promotion advice from pharmacists

The published work to date suggests on the one hand that consumers are broadly accepting of the idea of pharmacists providing health advice and will respond to pharmacy health promotion campaigns. On the other hand, few would take the initiative in approaching the pharmacist and asking for advice, and the pharmacist is not yet seen by the public as a source from which they would expect to receive general health advice. A 1996 RPSGB survey of the general population showed that only 11 per cent had *sought* general health advice from pharmacists, and that half of these were seeking advice about medicine usage. This advice-seeking group consisted mainly of women, people with children, those in lower social classes (C2DE), and 'striving' and inner city respondents. Overall, 14 per cent of respondents reported that they had received unsolicited health-related advice in the pharmacy (defined by the researchers as seeing a poster, picking up a leaflet, or if the pharmacist had spoken to them about a particular health-related product or issue). Such advice had been received twice on average in the last year and was more likely to have been received by respondents with children and by heavier users of pharmacies. These findings, although not generalizable, suggest that pharmacy health promotion activity should target more resources to these sectors of the population who use the pharmacy most.

In the evaluation of the Barnet scheme, people with prescriptions were more likely than others to regard the pharmacist as someone to go to for advice about staying healthy. Those Barnet consumers who had taken health promotion leaflets were significantly more likely to be those who had asked the pharmacist about general health and those who thought it was the 'usual job' of the pharmacists to give health advice. These, in turn, were more likely to be regular prescription customers. These findings suggest that if pharmacists are to reach the healthy population who are not yet receiving prescriptions, new strategies will be needed.

Another important issue is that of privacy in the pharmacy, and consumer surveys have shown consistently that about half of those asked say that there is insufficient privacy. Creative design of consultation areas means that it is feasible to create such areas in even small pharmacies.

Consumer surveys also show that the public's perception is that the pharmacist is always busy in the dispensary and it is likely that, as a result, many people may be inhibited from asking directly for the pharmacist's advice.

5.2   What is the pharmacist's role?

5.2.1   Defining the role

Health promotion is something that all pharmacists can be involved in and indeed is one of the key areas identified in the Royal

Pharmaceutical Society's 'Pharmacy in a New Age' strategy. In recent years, many pharmacists have changed their attitude towards health promotion and now accept it as an important part of pharmacy practice, although perhaps not yet as a core activity. This is understandable when most of the pharmacy's income comes from dispensing NHS prescriptions and where remuneration for health promotion other than for 'pilot' projects is rare.

To be taken seriously as health promoters, pharmacists must show that they can produce health gain in a cost-effective manner. Health promotion is not just about changing lifestyle, nor is it about simply providing information. It is also about providing services that improve the health of individuals and communities and empowering people to have increased control over and to improve their health.

5.2.2 Activity levels in health promotion

Health promotion can occur at different levels and might depend on how well the pharmacist knows particular patients and customers. All pharmacists can provide a basic service, and many can do more. The most basic involvement is through the leaflets that community pharmacies are required to display to qualify for the professional allowance. The pharmacist's involvement can range from passive to active including:

- Passive display of leaflets
- Pro-active use of leaflets in response to requests for advice
- Pro-active use of leaflets in opportunistic advice-giving.

Pharmacists can do far more to promote health by using the premises and other pharmacy resources, including their own influencing skills:

- Use of the pharmacy premises and environment to promote health messages (window displays, in-store displays)
- Using patient medication records to target specific patient groups and offer health-related advice (for example about exercise and nutrition for patients receiving medicines for hypertension)
- Collaborating with local medical practices in promoting uptake of vaccination and screening programmes

- Providing health promotion clinics in the pharmacy or medical practice (for example on smoking cessation, menopause)
- Active participation by the pharmacist in lobbying for health change locally and nationally.

Two levels of health promotion were proposed in the Royal Pharmaceutical Society's 1998 *'Guidance for the development of health promotion by community pharmacists'* and are shown in Box 5.1. Level one would be expected for all pharmacists and level two for those who wished to specialize.

Recognizing that not all pharmacists will wish to work at level two, it is important to identify the kinds of activities that might reasonably be expected at level one (see Box 5.2).

Box 5.1   The two levels of pharmacist involvement in health promotion (RPSGB, 1998)

Level one (generalist)

Focuses on the pharmacist encouraging healthy behaviour. The pharmacist will set aside an area in the pharmacy for health promotion literature and information. Pharmacists and their trained staff will use leaflets to highlight health issues. Simple health promotion advice will be given when handing out prescriptions, making sales, and advising about treating symptoms.

Level two (specialist and pro-active)

In addition to level one activities, the pharmacist actively seeks opportunities to promote health. If appropriate, they will identify the stage of change person is at for the particular behaviour and offer individualized advice and ongoing support.

Box 5.2   Expected activities for all pharmacists (level one)

- present medicines in a way that helps to prevent accidents in the home
- take part in campaigns for the disposal of unwanted medicines
- give health promotion advice linked to the sale and supply of medicines
- give health promotion advice linked to presenting symptoms
- utilize information leaflets and other health promotion materials appropriately
- take part in local and national health promotion events
- give simple dietary advice in response to requests for advice about symptoms where dietary factors are relevant (e.g. constipation, indigestion)
- give simple advice on smoking cessation and promote the use of nicotine replacement therapy
- give advice on request about contraception and safe sex, conception, pregnancy, breast feeding, immunization and health of under-5's
- give evidence-based health promotion advice
- take part in a needle exchange scheme and a supervised methadone administration scheme, if appropriate

---

Pharmacists should work towards health gain and not just lifestyle changes, aiming to improve the health of the people they come into contact with, helping to increase the number of years that people spend free of illness. An understanding of the socio-economic position of the pharmacy's patients and customers is an important pre-requisite. Pharmacists in deprived areas see the worst off in society and can help to tackle inequalities in health. Research has shown that pharmacies are used by those in the lower social classes (C2DE) and 'striving' and inner city respondents. The philosophy and skills needed for health promotion are similar to those necessary for concordance (see Chapter 6).

Beattie's structural grid (see Fig. 5.1) presents a taxonomy of health promotion that attempts to incorporate the spectrum of activities that might be conducted. The framework identifies four discrete areas of health promotion:

1. *Health persuasion*—interventions directed at individuals led by professionals, e.g. a pharmacist encouraging a pregnant woman to stop smoking.

2. *Legislative action*—interventions led by professionals intended to protect individuals, e.g. pharmacists lobbying parliament to make nicotine replacement therapy available on prescription.

3. *Personal counselling*—interventions led by individuals; the health promoter acts as a facilitator not an expert, e.g. pharmacist-led smoking cessation clinics for individuals.

4. *Community development*—interventions such as those in personal counselling, seeking to empower a group or a local community, e.g. a community group asks the pharmacist to set up a smoking cessation clinic.

The grid provides a means of comparing the different philosophies of health promoters through analysis of the quadrant where their work originates.

Traditionally, pharmacists have adopted the role of expert, instructing their customers and providing factual information. A model of practice involving counselling and negotiation has not generally been the pharmacist's usual way of working. However, the research evidence on approaches most likely to be acceptable to users and more likely to be effective shows that the Stages of Change model (Chapter 4) and the concept of concordance (see Chapter 6) should be adopted more widely by pharmacists. These approaches fit most closely with quadrant 3 of Beattie's framework. The framework was used to examine pharmacists' health promotion activities in the evaluation of the Barnet scheme. On the whole, and despite their training, which explored the wider context of health promotion, pharmacists worked from a model where the pharmacist is the expert persuading people to change. This finding suggests that pharmacists might find it difficult to adopt a style of working in which the customer's views and decisions are of equal value. There are important implications both for the extent to which pharmacists engage in health promotion and for the effectiveness of pharmacists' inputs. Education and training, beginning at undergraduate level, will be needed to achieve change.

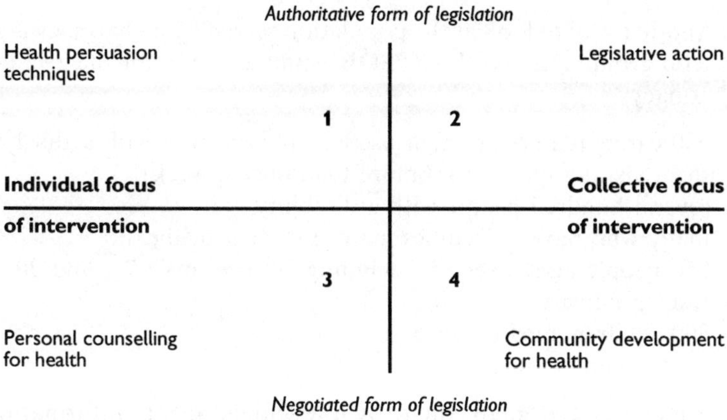

Authoritative form of legislation

Health persuasion techniques		Legislative action
	1	**2**
Individual focus		**Collective focus**
of intervention		**of intervention**
	3	**4**
Personal counselling for health		Community development for health

Negotiated form of legislation

Fig. 5.1 Strategies of health promotion (Beattie, 1990).

5.3 The pharmacy setting

5.3.1 Understanding the pharmacy's clientele

An understanding of the clientele of the pharmacy is important in thinking about the kinds of health promotion activity that might be undertaken. In the early 1990s, the Royal Pharmaceutical Society estimated that an 'average' pharmacy might expect to serve:

- up to 500 people taking antihypertensive medication
- 150 asthmatics
- 50 diabetics,
- eight people with colostomies
- three people with coeliac disease
- 20 people suffering from cancer (of which four will be receiving palliative care)
- at least two people who have AIDS or are HIV positive
- a range of drug users

- one person with cystic fibrosis,
- several people who are keen to stop taking tranquillisers
- a small number of people with chronic mental health problems
- 15 people discharged from hospital in the last week (including day surgery patients)

Another way to look at the population served by a pharmacy is at general groupings, and the RPSGB estimates were, for the average pharmacy:

- 600 carers (carers are high users of pharmacies, with a third of them visiting pharmacies more than once a week)
- several hundred people with a disability
- many who have difficulties managing their medication
- 750 people aged over 65, including 30 aged over 75, and 20 in residential care
- 300 children aged under 5
- 50 pregnant women

Pharmacists can map their own clientele using information resources such as their patient medication records so that they can target their activities more effectively.

5.3.2   Effect of the pharmacy premises

Another aspect of the pharmacy setting that needs to be considered is whether it promotes or acts as a barrier to health promotion. Firstly, physical barriers to access need to be addressed by providing ramps for wheelchair access and a layout suitable for disabled, pushchairs, and so on.

Health-promoting pharmacies should have a professional atmosphere, a consulting area, and space for the display of health promotion information. Information should be accessible and signposted. Leaflet racks, display boards, and window displays should be updated regularly. Links for referral to the primary health care team and other agencies, for example self-help groups, drugs workers, and social services, should be made through networking by the pharmacist, and directories for local and national referral should be available in the pharmacy to put customers in touch with the most relevant local or national contacts.

Pharmacists need to reflect on the product ranges that are stocked, and keep those that positively promote health, while not stocking those which could be detrimental to health. Examples would be not stocking sweets, or sugar-containing weaning products. The product range should reflect the needs of the local area, for example stocking a wide range of mobility aids may not be appropriate where most customers were young mothers. To be credible as a source of smoking cessation advice, the pharmacy needs to have a no smoking policy.

Pharmacists have been criticized because they are operating in an overtly commercial environment. However, their accessibility rivals that of any other health care providers and the public are increasingly willing to consult pharmacists about health matters. Pharmacy window campaigns have shown, for example, that when the public are made aware that pharmacists can give advice on matters such as emergency contraception, diabetes, and stroke the public will ask many more questions about these issues than normal.

Some pharmacies will become healthy living centres, for example pharmacies in Alfreton (South Derbyshire) and Lanarkshire have been developed as a health information centre and a health-promoting pharmacy, respectively. Other examples of using the pharmacy setting include a women's health afternoon held by the Tesco pharmacy in Huddersfield. The event was attended by 45 women, with a very positive response. Pharmacists from Boots the Chemists at Monument, City of London ran lunch-time talks at Lloyds of London in conjunction with the Lloyds' occupational health team. Talks were given on general health issues pertinent to the audience on 'how to survive the party season' and 'spring cleaning your first aid box'.

5.3.3 Remuneration

An important part of the community pharmacy setting is an understanding of the relationship between remuneration and activity. Research with pharmacists shows consistently that lack of remuneration for health promotion work is a barrier to its greater provision. The NHS contract funds the dispensing of prescriptions on a 'per item' basis and, for those pharmacies dispensing sufficient prescriptions to qualify for it, a professional allowance payment. The latter includes a component for the display of specified health promotion leaflets, agreed locally. Funding for health promotion schemes has therefore had to come from other sources, and has often been from health authorities.

Consumers themselves might be expected to pay for particular services, and some pharmacists have established self-funding initiatives. Terry Maguire, a community pharmacy health promotion innovator in Northern Ireland, developed a pharmacy smoking cessation advice service in his Belfast pharmacy. Customers were charged £25 to enrol in a service that involved an initial interview and regular follow up; customers also purchased nicotine replacement therapy where appropriate. However, given that those most in need of health promotion are likely to be those who can least afford to pay for it, the scope for consumer payments is likely to be variable depending on the socio-economic circumstances of the pharmacy customers.

5.4   The future—emerging infrastructure for the pharmacist's contribution to health promotion

Health Improvement Programmes (HImPs) and their equivalents will provide the outline for health promotion until at least 2005. Pharmacists need to ensure that they at least have a copy of their local HImP and ideally will find a way to contribute to its development. Collaborative working will be key—with health authorities/health boards; primary care groups and equivalents; local health promotion specialist units; other professional groups; and local authorities.

5.4.1   Health authority/Health board-sponsored activities

Many health authorities have supported and funded local pharmacy-based health promotion schemes, although resources have often been limited. A 1994 survey of health authorities showed that one of the most frequently mentioned barriers to developing health promotion activities for community pharmacists was lack of financial resources. Another major factor was lack of pharmaceutical advisers' time for community pharmacy development. Schemes appear to have been more successful when the Local Pharmaceutical Committee, local specialist health promotion services, and others such as primary care development managers have been jointly involved in their implementation.

In a 1997 survey, smoking cessation was the most popular subject for pharmacy-based health promotion events sponsored by health authorities. Other subjects included sun safety, folic acid, minor ailments, emergency contraception, mental health, and oral health. Examples of specific projects are shown below in Box 5.3

Box 5.3   Examples of health authority-sponsored pharmacy health promotion projects

- Avon health authority evaluated the feasibility of promoting physical activity from community pharmacies.
- Southampton and South West Hampshire health authority worked with the Royal National Institute for the Blind to increase referrals to optometrists for sight tests.
- St Helen's and Knowsley health authority trained pharmacists in advising patients about medicines for heart conditions and healthy living, and paid six community pharmacists to provide clinics in GP surgeries.
- East Yorkshire health authority trained six community pharmacists in one locality to provide advice about stopping smoking. Customers who asked for advice about or present prescriptions for contraception, asthma, or coronary heart disease were issued with a tracking card and could ask for advice in any of the six pharmacies. A campaign on folic acid was planned.
- South Staffordshire trained 13 community pharmacists and paid them to provide a health promotion service based on the Stages of Change model, with a brief interview and

clients invited back for a longer discussion where needed. The areas to be covered in the first year were oral health, increasing physical activity, improving diet, and smoking cessation.

- West Glamorgan's pharmacy health promotion scheme began in 1994 and had a focus on securing standards in the pharmacy setting to support health promotion activities. Pharmacists were provided with health promotion resources but not remuneration. Local advertising and press coverage were used to publicize the scheme. Protocols were developed for oral health, smoking cessation, and communicable diseases/infestations.

5.4.2 Primary care groups

Traditional professional roles are being redefined, and the development of primary care groups (PCGs) in England and their equivalents in other countries will change this further. The role of the pharmacist in medicines management is likely to move higher up the primary care agenda. A recent study concluded that pharmacists can play a strategic role in keeping minor illness out of general practice. Management of a greater proportion of episodes of minor illness by pharmacists could alter GPs' workload, increasing the time that they have available to deal with those who really need a GP consultation. GPs are often unaware of the training that pharmacists now receive in diagnosing minor illness and distinguishing it from major disease. GPs are sometimes reluctant to delegate, fearing that other health care professionals will miss a serious diagnosis, although there is little evidence to support this view. Joint training is a good way of breaking down some of these barriers, and the use of protocols can implement agreed and shared approaches and treatments.

The traditional settings of where pharmacists practice are also changing, for example more GP surgeries and PCGs are employing pharmacists to work as advisers. To date, these primary care pharmacists (PCPs) have been involved predominantly in providing prescribing advice and medication review clinics, although their role in health promotion may develop in the future. High street pharmacies might have a greater role in the future as health advice centres. The benefits of team working should be integration, enhanced patient care, and improved health outcomes through, for example, the development of shared guidance, referral protocols, ownership, and commitment.

5.4.3 Local specialist health promotion services

Specialist health promotion services may be located in health authorities, NHS trusts, or in agencies within health authorities. They are responsible for the provision of expert advice, training, and resources to support local health promotion activity and are an essential contact. They liaise with other local and national health promotion agencies to ensure that activities are coordinated and supported. Health promotion services often provide resources (such as leaflets) for use in health promotion events. They have been involved in a large number of training initiatives for pharmacists and their staff.

5.4.4 Other professional groups

Health promotion will often involve different professionals and disciplines working together, for example pharmacists might work with the local GP practice, a community nurse, a health visitor, a midwife, a local dental practice, local optician, an environmental health officer, and so on. The National Pharmaceutical Association and the PHS have piloted a smoking cessation service package to be used jointly in GP surgeries and community pharmacies.

Multidisciplinary training is in its infancy, although a number of health promotion units provide some mixed training that pharmacists have attended. Further moves here are important, and pharmacists should be involved in training other health care professionals so that they will begin to understand the role of the pharmacist in health promotion. *Our Healthier Nation* encourages joint training in health promotion.

Ealing Hammersmith and Hounslow health authority have funded joint training of nurses and community pharmacists to be coronary heart disease facilitators. The facilitators encourage local nurses, pharmacists, and GPs to give consistent advice and to share information.

The development of HAZs will encourage working with local authorities and closer links between health and social care. Croydon pharmacists, in conjunction with the local authority, were the first in the country to be involved in a scheme to display information on social services in their pharmacies.

5.5   Realizing the potential of community pharmacists as health promoters—the challenges that remain

The major arguments put forward to legitimize the pharmacist's role in health promotion are:

- The opportunities which the pharmacy setting offers both for provision of information and through the direct input of the pharmacist
- Community pharmacists are available for at least 8 and for up to 14 hours a day without an appointment
- They see the healthy as well as the ill
- Their position on the high street enables their premises to be used for health promotion campaigns which will reach a large number of people
- The relationship that a pharmacist builds up with patients, customers, and their families over years, and its essentially informal nature (in contrast to that with the GP)
- Users have a free choice of pharmacy and can seek advice at any pharmacy they wish
- Pharmacists potentially can make a large contribution to local campaigns and reinforce the messages being given in GPs' surgeries, clinics, hospitals, and 'one-stop health shops'.

All of these are powerful and persuasive arguments. However, as we have seen earlier in this chapter, a number of challenges remain.

- Pharmacists need to move towards a style of practice which involves negotiation rather than 'telling', and which recognizes the individual's decisions and choices

- Health promotion needs to become a 'way of thinking and working' for pharmacists rather than an 'add-on' activity
- The accessibility of community pharmacists without appointment may be feasible for brief interventions but not for longer ones
- Prescription customers are more likely to seek and accept general health advice from the pharmacist. Pharmacists need to be seen as more general health advisers, and changing the perceptions of the non-prescription and healthy consumers currently poses more of a challenge.
- Consumers perceive that the pharmacist is always busy, and may be reluctant to ask to speak to the pharmacist. Greater use of dispensing technicians would create more time for pharmacists to spend directly with the public.
- More pharmacists need to create space for confidential conversations. The inclusion of consultation areas in pharmacies is an important step in creating the greater privacy which many consumers want to have.

For pharmacy to move forward in its health promotion role, ways need to be found and tested to address these challenges.

References

Beattie, A. (1984) Health education and the science teacher: an invitation to debate. *Education and health* 1, 9–16.

Beattie, A. (1990) Knowledge and control in health promotion. In Gabe, J., Calman, M., and Bury, M. *Sociology of the Health Service*. Routledge, Kegan and Paul, London.

Prochaska, J. and DiClemente, C. (1982) Transtheoretical therapy— towards a more integrative model of change. *Psychotherapy: theory, research and practice* 19, 276–88.

Table 5.1 Development of health promotion in community pharmacy

Date	Health promotion*	Date	Health promotion in pharmacy
1900	Concern for infant and child health: health visitors, mother and baby clinics, school medical service	1900	Pharmacists advising patients and dispensing medicines
1906–14	Liberal Government reforms, National Insurance and Old Age Pensions	1908	
1919	Ministry of Health and numerous voluntary organizations produce leaflets and posters		
1927	Central Council for Health Education of Medical Officers of Health, Local Authority Associations and Health Insurance Committees		
1940–4	Major campaigns, e.g. to promote diphtheria immunization, venereal disease education		
1946	Responsibility for health education transferred to Local Authorities		
1948	NHS started	1948	Pharmacists concentrate more on dispensing NHS prescriptions
1957	First training courses for health education specialists at London University Institute of Education.	1964	First report of pharmacists involvement—dental health campaign in west of Scotland
1968	First health education officers appointed by Local Authorities Health Education Council (HEC) funded by Department of Health and Social Security (DHSS)	1965	Mearns—pharmacists have a vital role to play in health education. Aldington—should display health education literature
		1968	Call for pharmacy representation on HEC
1970s	High profile mass media campaigns on smoking, immunization, and family planning. Support for curriculum work in schools, support for training and research. Prochaska and diClemente start to develop and test the 'Stages of Change' model	1970	Conference on role of pharmacist in health education
		1973	William Darling, first pharmacist to serve on HEC
		1978	Working group on general practice pharmacy say that health education including diagnostic testing important

1976	NHS reorganization, creation of Community Health Councils	1980s	Research into pharmacist role in health promotion begins, notably Harris in South East Thames and Panton in West Midlands
1976	*Prevention and health everybody's business* published by the DHSS—concentrated on a behavioural approach which sees health problems as a result of individual lifestyles followed by numerous reports on prevention	1986	Healthcare in the High Street launched
		1986	*Nuffield Report*—role for community pharmacists in health education in cooperation with other health professionals, review remuneration in light of increasing professional role
1977	WHO declaration at Alma Ata committing members to the principles of health for all 2000	1986	Brent and Harrow Family Practitioner Committee say they will support health education role of pharmacist
1982	Reorganization of the NHS—District Health Authorities. Publication of the *Black Report* on inequalities in health	1987	Promoting Better Health 'pharmacists can make an important contribution to health promotion—funds for Healthcare in the High Street Scheme
1984	*Griffiths Report*, general managers to run NHS instead of health professionals	1987	Work on health promotion begins in Northern Ireland—Morrow *et al.* on education, Maguire *et al.* on health screening
1987	*Promoting Better Health* White Paper, GPs encouraged to carry out health promotion linked to financal incentives for health checks and reaching targeted vaccination levels	1987	Pharmacists consider their role in health education in the light of AIDS and HIV
1987	HEA superseded HEC	1990	FHSAs formed, pharmaceutical advisers appointed, interest in community pharmacy development. Discussions on health promotion undergraduate curriculum
1987	Ottawa Charter for Health Promotion signed		
1988	Focus on the issues of AIDS and HIV and drug misuse receive large sums of money major advertising first AIDS awareness campaign	1991	Barnet FHSA High Street Health Scheme launched Discussions on pharmacists' role in the light of the *Health of the Nation*
1988	Look After Your Heart campaign launched to raise awareness of coronary heart disease	1992	*Acheson Report* on public health in England
1990	*Acheson Report* on public health in England	1993–4	Pharmacy Healthcare Scheme established as a charity
1990	NHS and Community Care Act divided NHS up into purchaser and provider units		
1992	New GP contract introduces targets and payments for health promotion		

Table 5.1 (cont.)

Date	Health promotion*	Date	Health promotion in pharmacy
1992	The *Health of the Nation* White Paper published in England (and equivalents in Scotland/Wales/ Northern Ireland)	1994	*Pharmaceutical Care Report*—role in health promotion and diagnostic testing
1998	*Our Healthier Nation* green paper published (and equivalents in Scotland/Wales/Northern Ireland)	1994	Professional allowance includes health promotion leaflet requirement
1998	*Smoking Kills* White Paper published	1994	Nearly two-thirds of FHSAs report pharmacy health promotion activity
		1994	Launch of the Pharmacists Against Smoking (PAS) initiative based on Stages of Change model
		1996	*Primary Care: The Future*—innovations in pharmacy health promotion be developed nationally
		1996	*Pharmacy in a New Age*—summary of responses— health promotion ranked as second most important role that should be expanded
		1998	Expert group report—Development of health promotion in community pharmacy commissioned by RPSGB

*History of health promotion from Naidoo and Wills (1994)

6 Concordance in medicine-taking

Treatment with medicines is an important component of promoting health. Yet it has been estimated that overall, patients' compliance with medicines is only around 50 per cent. The term 'concordance' describes an agreement between patient and health professional about what action is to be taken. Concordance is based on the principle that patients receive the information that they want and need about their medicines and can therefore decide on an informed basis. Central to concordance is an acceptance that an informed patient may decide they do not wish to take the treatment. Pharmacists and other health professionals need to accept that this may sometimes be the outcome. As the health professionals most involved with medicines, pharmacists have a key role to play in concordance. In this chapter, we will explore what the terms concordance and compliance mean, what patients want to know about their medicines, and how pharmacists can contribute to concordance.

6.1 The difference between compliance and concordance

The term 'compliance' has been used traditionally to describe 'the extent to which the patient follows the doctor's instructions'. Compliance therefore refers to the patient's behaviour in relation to their medicines. Over 20 years ago, a review of research found that 'rates of compliance with different long-term medication regimens for different illnesses in different settings tend to converge to approximately 50 per cent'. Thus patients have been termed 'low', ' high', or 'problem' compliers. In recent years, the term has fallen out of favour because it is thought to be judgmental and to imply that patients should simply do as they are told. To be non-compliant with a medicine regime was seen as 'deviant' behaviour until social scientist researchers and the growing movement supporting individual rights pointed out that this was inappropriate and that the reasons why a patient may or may not take their medicines were complex.

The term 'adherence' was then introduced, as it was thought to be less judgmental, although some people argue that it is really no different from the old concept of compliance.

In the mid-1990s, a multi-disciplinary group comprising pharmacists, doctors, nurses, and social scientists came together to review the evidence on compliance and to try to determine a constructive way forward. That group developed the notion of 'concordance' as a way of moving attention away from a focus on holding patients entirely responsible for medicine-taking and away from criticizing patients for not doing as the health professional recommended.

The term 'compliance' often is still used as a way of describing whether the patient is taking their treatment, and relating only to the patient's behaviour. Concordance is where the patient and health professional (doctor, pharmacist, or nurse) agree on what they will do about the treatment. Rather than the professional simply telling the patient what to do, concordance is about a discussion that involves the patient, where the patient is the decision-maker. In some cases, the agreement might be that the patient does not take the medicine. Patients have the right to make an informed choice in relation to medicines or any other treatment. Pharmacists, who have spent their training learning about the benefits of medicines, often see their role as persuading, cajoling, and generally influencing patients to follow the prescribed instructions. Like other health professionals, pharmacists may find it hard at first to accept that a patient may decline treatment. The reality is that currently many medicines are not taken, but health professionals are unaware in many cases that this is happening. Research has shown that health professionals are poor predictors of compliance among their patients. Concordance implies an open discussion about benefits and risks of treatment in which the patient has the opportunity to air their agenda and concerns. Thus concordance refers to the relationship between professional and patient and, by its nature, involves more than one person. Non-concordance would thus denote either a disagreement between patient and health professional, or a lack of discussion between them. Patients cannot themselves be 'concordant' or 'non-concordant', and this highlights the difference from the notion of compliance.

Working towards the goal of concordance will require a major shift in the way that health services are delivered, including more and longer consultations between patients and health professionals, more user-friendly information for patients, and a change in health professionals' stance to respect the autonomy of the patient.

6.2   Information—the gap between what patients want and what health professionals think they should receive

Despite the many changes that have taken place in the last 20 years —more effective medicines and more information for patients— there is no evidence that the issue of low compliance has been resolved. A review of research on interventions to improve compliance concluded in 1996 that 'effective ways to help people follow medical treatments would have far larger effects on health than any treatment itself'. However, one thing that most of these studies had in common was that the interventions were usually designed from the point of view of the health professionals rather than the patients. This meant that the information that was given, for example, was what health professionals thought patients should receive rather than being based on what the patients themselves wanted.

Research into patients' own ideas about medicines and about the information they would like to receive gives us some clues about 'the compliance problem'. Most people (about three-quarters) would like to receive more information than they currently do. Many of these people would like to be more involved in decisions about their treatment (Coulter, 1997). More detail on the information patients say they would like to receive about medicines is given later in this chapter on page 111.

6.3   Unintentional and intentional non-compliance

Patients' intent to take their medicines is the basis for standard definitions of compliance. In unintentional non-compliance, the patient's intent to take the treatment may be overcome by a variety of practical barriers. Intentional non-compliance is where the patient makes a conscious decision not to take the medicine, or to take it differently from the prescribed regime.

6.3.1 Unintentional non-compliance

Possible causes of unintentional non-compliance are shown in Table 6.1.

Like other health professionals, pharmacists generally feel more comfortable with unintentional non-compliance because there are various practical actions that can be taken to help patients overcome the barriers to medicine-taking.

Forgetfulness is an almost universal problem, particularly where the patient is taking a number of different medicines and the dosage schedule is complex. Research shows that reducing the number of daily doses of a medicine to one or two improves compliance compared with three or four times daily dosing. The evidence that once daily dosing is better than twice daily in this respect is not definitive.

Prompts and reminders

Research has shown that prompts and reminders can help. These can be visual, such as a Medicines Reminder Chart or Medicines Information Sheet (see Fig. 6.1), which has been shown to improve both knowledge and compliance. Such charts set out the times of day, with names of medicines and how much is to be taken. The chart can also include the purpose of each medicine. Medicines reminder charts are most useful for patients on many medicines with varying dose frequencies. Instead of having to look at all the bottle labels all the time, the patient simply looks at the chart. This tells them what they need to take at the four events given on the chart (usually breakfast, lunch-time, evening meal, and bedtime). It should be borne in mind that not all patients have three meals and it may be appropriate to substitute different daily events which suit that particular patient.

Another approach is the use of an alarm or physical reminder. A recent TV programme on pagers showed how they are used by spouses and relatives to remind patients to take their medicine.

Table 6.1. Unintentional non-compliance: practical difficulties and possible actions

Problem	Action
Lack of knowledge/ understanding about the disease/condition and its treatment	• Written information (Patient Information Leaflets—PILs) • Verbal information (reinforcing the information in the PIL)
Impaired sight	• Large print or braille labels • Let the patient tape your counselling or arrange for the PIL to be taped
Reduced manual dexterity	• Use non-CRC bottles • Check patient can cope with foil or blister packaging • Check patient can cope with measuring doses of liquids. If problems, consider dispensing in smaller (hence less heavy) bottles or solid dose form • For eye drops, check the patient can instil them. If problems, consider an eyedrop compliance aid (e.g. Autodrop)
Problems swallowing solid dose forms	• Suggest change to liquids or use of lower strength (likely to be smaller) tablets
Inability to use non-oral dose forms	• Check technique and arrange for a teaching session
Poor reading skills	• Concentrate on verbal counselling • Offer continuing information back-up on the telephone
Forgetting	• Full labelling with instructions—not 'as before' or as directed' • Suggest to GP that regimen is simplified • Prompts and reminders, e.g. Precise dose timing (breakfast, lunchtime, etc.) Reminder charts Pagers/alarms Telephone call Special containers Get relatives or carers to help
Side-effects	• Anticipate common side-effects • Encourage patients to report side-effects
Confusion over complex regime	• Offer a 'brown bag' session • Tailor regime to patient's lifestyle • Approach GP re rationalization of regime

Information about your medicines

Name: _____

Date: _____

How to use this chart

● This chart shows you when to take each of your medicines.

● At each meal time, look down the column to see which medicines you need to take **with or just after** the meal. Do the same about half an hour before bedtime.

● A spoon means a 5ml plastic medicine spoon.

● Medicines which you take only when you need them are **not** included in the chart.

Medicine	Breakfast	Lunch-time	Evening meal	Bed-time

If there is a * by the dose, this means you should take the medicine ½ to 1 hour before food.

Fig. 6.1 Medicines Reminder Card. (Source: National Pharmaceutical Association, tel. 01727 858687 ext. 469.)

A little extreme, some would think, but they can work well. Telephone calls can be used to remind patients when their next repeat prescription is due as well as to check how patients are getting on with their medicines.

Special containers such as monitored dosage systems have a place in helping some patients to organize their medicine doses, but should not be a first-line approach. Patients need to be assessed carefully for their ability to remove medicines from these containers. Other, simpler, approaches, should be tried first.

Visual impairment

Visual impairment is common, and research shows that community pharmacists tend to underestimate the extent to which this is a problem for their own patients. The use of large type labelling is helpful, and computerized patient medication records (PMRs) can be flagged to provide a prompt to provide them. Simple charts or instructions written in large lettering with a felt tip pen can be useful. Braille labels are also valuable, and it is important to note that not all patients who are registered blind can read braille—in fact the number who can do so is small.

Side-effects

Providing patients with information about side-effects has been controversial. In the past, many health professionals have tended to withhold information about side-effects due to understandable concerns that patients may become worried and stop taking their medicine, or even that they might imagine they were experiencing such effects when they were not. Research evidence shows, however, that patients prefer to know about side-effects and that compliance is not necessarily reduced by giving this information. When patients know the common minor side-effects that might occur, and what to do about them, they are more likely to continue treatment or to discuss with their doctor or pharmacist what to do next. However, where patients obtain information about side-effects that concerns them and they perceive difficulty in discussing this with a health professional, there may be a risk that their concerns remain unaddressed and one possibility is that the patient may stop taking the medicine. Patients work out their own risk–benefit analysis, and providing more information about side-effects may result in some patients making an informed decision not to take their medicine.

Contrary to the belief of many pharmacists, research shows that telling patients about possible side-effects does not mean that more patients will report such effects incorrectly or inappropriately. The only exception to this appears to be for benzodiazepines. The lengthy lists of side-effects found in patient information leaflets can be alarming to patients, but it is likely that this is because there is often little differentiation between common and rare effects. This is an area where the pharmacist can interpret and explain the information. In the longer term, the increased use of consumer testing in the development of patient information leaflets should make them more patient-friendly.

6.3.2 Intentional non-compliance

Intentional non-compliance is where the patient makes a deliberate decision not to take the medicine or to alter their dosage schedule without consultation with the doctor. The latter is sometimes referred to as self-regulation of dosing. Pharmacists and other health professionals often find intentional non-compliance more difficult to understand and accept. The examples below illustrate some of the reasons why patients make decisions and choices about their medicines.

Case 1: Dave, a 25-year-old man, was prescribed fluoxetine for his depression. He was worried that he would become addicted to the medicine, or that he would need to depend on it forever, because he had once read that tranquilisers were addictive. So he stopped taking it after a month. However, he saw the GP and had a repeat prescription dispensed because he did not want the doctor to think he was ungrateful or ignoring her advice. The GP assumed he had taken the medicine and that his depression had resolved. The pharmacist assumed he was taking the tablets and that the doctor had stopped the treatment after 3 months.

Case 2: Jane, a 52-year-old woman, stopped taking her HRT after 3 months because she was experiencing irregular bleeding and thought this meant the medicine was causing a serious problem that would be worse than her menopausal symptoms. She did not discuss this with her doctor. The pharmacist noticed from the PMR that she no longer received the treatment, but assumed the doctor had decided to discontinue it.

Case 3: Ray, a 58-year-old man, had only ever taken part of his dose of imipramine because he found the side-effects intolerable. In particular, he was worried about the effect his tiredness might have on his driving. When his depression got worse, his doctor increased the dose of imipramine but Ray felt unable to tell him that he had not been taking the full amount previously and felt there was no way he could take any more. His depression became worse. The GP thought he had solved the problem by increasing the dose. The pharmacist noted from the PMR that the dose had gone up and thought that since the patient had been receiving imipramine for a long time there was no need for any advice or information.

Case 4: Edith, a 90-year-old lady, only took her analgesics (Co-codamol) when the pain was 'really bad' because she thought her body would 'get used' to them and they would not work when she 'really needed them'. As a result, she put up with pain on a daily basis. Her kitchen cupboard had many bottles of unused analgesic because she regularly collected her supply. She rarely saw the GP, who was not aware that she was in pain. The 'as directed' instructions and collection of regular repeats led the pharmacist to believe that Edith was getting the relief from pain that she needed.

Case 5: Sara, a 24-year-old woman with asthma, collected her repeat prescription for salbutamol and beclomethasone inhalers as regular as clockwork. But she never used the beclomethasone because she had heard it was a steroid and had terrible side-effects. In any case, she believed that she only had a 'chest problem' and not asthma—people with asthma were much worse than her. She felt better and healthier if she could cope without the inhaled steroid. However, she was taking a herbal remedy for her asthma because she felt it was 'natural'. No one at the GP surgery ever asked her how she was using the two inhalers. From the pharmacy PMRs, she appeared to be a 'fully compliant' patient.

Case 6: Jane, a 59-year-old woman, stopped taking the HRT her doctor had prescribed to prevent osteoporosis after 3 years because her sister had died of breast cancer. She had read in a newspaper that HRT could cause breast cancer and she thought she might get it too. Ten years later, she was admitted to hospital with a fractured femur because she had developed osteoporosis. At her repeat prescription review, it was not noticed that she had not been requesting the HRT. The pharmacist assumed the doctor had stopped the treatment.

Case 7: Roy, a 45-year-old man, was diagnosed with hypertension. After a few months, the doctor doubled the dose of his antihypertensive medication. Roy started going to the gym, became fitter and lost weight. He started to feel dizzy and faint sometimes and decided to change the dose of his tablets back to the original amount. Next time he saw the GP he did not mention this, but the GP commented that his blood pressure was 'normal'. Roy did not tell him about the change in dose. The pharmacist's PMR showed that Roy was collecting his prescription too infrequently for the prescribed dose to be taken, but this was not noticed either.

Box 6.1 shows some possible reasons for intentional non-compliance. As we saw in Chapter 4, patients often make their own, sometimes sophisticated risk–benefit analyses of certain behaviours, and medicine-taking is no exception to this.

Box 6.1   Possible causes of intentional non-compliance

- Denial of the diagnosis
- Patient's risk–benefit analysis not in favour of medicine-taking
- Medicine-taking places restrictions on lifestyle (e.g. where alcohol intake needs to be reduced)
- Differences in beliefs between patient and health professional (e.g. patient believes antidepressants to be addictive)

Table 6.2 shows how patients' health beliefs might affect their use of medicines.

The reason why the concept of concordance is so important is that it requires discussion between patient and health professional that is different from the kinds of interactions that often happen now. Health professionals sometimes are surprised to find that many patients have their own ideas and explanations for what is going wrong with the body in various conditions. These ideas might be quite different from health professionals' own explana-

Table 6.2 Influence of health beliefs on the use of medicines

Health belief	Explanation	Examples
Perceived efficacy	The patient's view on whether the medicine will work	Belief that branded medicines work better than generics Belief that prescribed medicines are 'stronger' than OTCs
Possibility of becoming 'immune' to the medicine's effects	The belief that if a medicine is taken regularly it will become less effective	Antibiotics; painkillers
'Unnaturalness' of manufactured medicines	The view that 'natural' therapies are safer and better	Discontinuing 'modern' medicines in favour of herbal and homoeopathic medicines
Danger of addiction and dependence	Worry about not being able to stop taking or do without the medicine	Antidepressants; painkillers
Anti-drug attitude	Equating medicines with drugs of abuse	Belief that inhaled steroids are the same as the steroids abused by body-builders
Balancing risks and benefits	The patient's own calculations and trade-offs of perceived risks and benefits	Parents' concerns about the effects of inhaled steroids on their child's growth
Managing everyday life	Belief that people should be able to control 'social' problems without resorting to medicines Belief that certain problems are 'natural' and should not be medicalized	Reluctance to take antidepressants and anxiolytics Reluctance to use HRT for menopausal symptoms

Adapted from patient belief themes identified by Dr Nicky Britten (Britten 1994).

tions, and are sometimes termed 'common-sense' explanations. In hypertension, for example, research shows that patients do not necessarily see this condition as being the same as high blood pressure. Some patients believe the condition to be literally a state of high stress or tension and that treatment works by reducing stress in some way. It is not difficult to see that such patients might adjust the dose of their medication in relation to their perceived level of stress.

6.4   What patients want to know about their medicines

Most patients (research findings indicate probably over three-quarters) would like to receive more information about medicines than they currently do. However, research also shows that patients and health professionals have different priorities for information about medicines. Patients need to know about both their disease or condition and their treatment. Pharmacists often assume that the doctor will have discussed the disease with the patient, but research suggests that patients either do not receive this information, or they cannot recall it. Given what we know about recall of verbal information it is not surprising that patients may not be able to remember being given certain information, especially if this was during a consultation where the patient was worried or feeling stressed.

Pharmacists need to check what the patient has already been told and what else they would like to know. Box 6.2 shows the basic information patients themselves would most like to receive.

However, it would be simplistic to assume that simply providing information will change behaviour, as we have seen in Chapter 4. Indeed, this has been described as one of the 'great myths about compliance'. An understanding of patients' beliefs about medicines can help pharmacists to enter a discussion with the individual in a non-judgemental way. The questions below can be used to open the discussion and encourage patients to share their thoughts and concerns.

- How are you getting on with your medicines?
- Are you having any problems with them? (Follow up verbal and non-verbal signs)

- Do you think you are having any side-effects from your medicines?
- Is there anything about your medicines that you would like to know?
- Is there anything about your illness/condition that you would like to know?

Written information is an important back-up to the verbal information which the pharmacist gives to the patient since much of that will be forgotten. Information leaflets are thus a central plank of information support.

Box 6.2   Information patients want to receive about their medicines and their condition

- Why have I got this condition/disease and what causes it?
- Can it be cured?
- What is this medicine for; what does it do and what common side-effects does it have?
- How long will I have to take this treatment?
- How will the medicine fit in with my lifestyle?

6.4.1   The role of Patient Information Leaflets (PILs)

It is now a legal requirement that manufacturers include a PIL with their medicines. The scope of such leaflets is defined by law and it has been argued that in the past PILs have been more about avoiding litigation than providing the information that patients want. In addition, it has been argued that there is an imbalance of information, with more about risks than benefits. New EC guidelines are likely to have the effect of making PILs more patient-friendly by requiring consumer testing. The leaflets will be tested with healthy consumers of the appropriate age group who might be part of the target patient group. Such testing assesses consumers' ability to use the leaflet in two ways: finding pieces of information in the leaflet, and demonstrating understanding (by repeating key pieces of information in their own words). The leaflet producer would be required to show that 16 of 20 consumers can find and describe 15 key points in the leaflet.

Giving patients a PIL (including side-effects) has been shown to increase knowledge and patient satisfaction but not compliance. It is important to note that the research conducted was with leaflets which were considerably shorter than the new EC-style leaflets and which were handed directly to the patient rather than being in the medicine package. Thus the generalizability of the findings needs to be tested on newer leaflets and in the way in which they will be used in practice. Efficacy of leaflets depends on design, layout, and method of delivery, as well as the actual words used. Nevertheless, the PIL can be a useful start to a discussion where the pharmacist can begin to find out what the patient's needs and concerns are. The PIL inside the medicine pack is becoming the key patient information resource associated with a medicine. An important advantage of such leaflets is that all health professionals can access the information the patient is getting (through the PIL compendium published by the Association of the British Pharmaceutical Industry, ABPI). If the doctor, pharmacist, and nurse all base the verbal information they give on the manufacturer's PIL, then the patient will not receive conflicting messages.

The pharmacist can go through the leaflet with the patient, using it as an aide memoire. This will also help to show the patient that this is an important, relevant, and useful piece of information and worth reading in more detail.

Finally, in this chapter we will consider some of the key areas from *Our Healthier Nation* and issues in concordance. Pharmacists can consider bringing together advice on both medicines and lifestyle in these areas. Using PMRs to identify patients who could benefit from health promotion advice is a good starting point.

6.5   Coronary heart disease and stroke

This is an area where the purpose of treatment may be prevention of future ill-health and where the patient may not see immediate benefit from the medicine. Generally, where a condition is symptomatic and the treatment aims to reduce those symptoms (for example angina), it is understandable that the patient is likely to be more motivated to take it. For asymptomatic conditions and their treatments, this may not be the case. The main examples here are antihypertensives, lipid-lowering drugs, anticoagulants, and anti-platelet agents. Patients are expected to take antihypertensive or lipid-lowering drugs or aspirin on the basis that a stroke or heart attack might be prevented at some time in the future. Health professionals generally are convinced by the evidence that taking such medicines is a 'good thing'. The patient's perspective looks a little different—years of having to remember to take a medicine, being labelled as 'at risk', and perhaps suffering side-effects and feeling worse when taking the medicine than they did before. The pharmacist can use the frameworks given earlier in this chapter to give the patient the information they want, and to accept the patient's right to know about risks as well as benefits of treatment.

Another important area is secondary prevention following a myocardial infarction (MI). Here, patients may be motivated by the desire to prevent another heart attack. However, they need to receive appropriate information about the reason why the treatment has been prescribed. The health service's 'National Service Framework on Coronary Heart Disease' aims to encourage the uptake of aspirin, lipid-lowering drugs, and beta-blockers post-MI. Pharmacists have a key role to play here, especially in relation to aspirin, which is often purchased over the counter as this is cheaper than paying the prescription charge. Research shows that some people are taking daily aspirin for primary prevention without prior discussion with their doctor. Pharmacists can identify these cases and help to ensure aspirin is not taken by the minority of patients in whom the possible risks outweigh the benefits.

6.6   Mental health

Many of the drugs used to treat schizophrenia have serious and very unpleasant side-effects. Nevertheless, patients are expected to take them, and it is unsurprising that compliance is a problem. There have been several highly publicized cases where patients have stopped taking their medicines and have become violent as a result. Although such cases are in fact very rare, they highlight the difficulties in monitoring treatment. Pharmacists are in a position sometimes to know when a patient has not collected a supply of their treatment, and the ethical dilemma arises of whether this information should be passed on. With the development of patient care plans and with the patient's agreement, there can be an agreement for pharmaceutical care that the pharmacist will let the appropriate person (for example the community mental health nurse or GP) know if the medicines have not been collected. They can then arrange to visit the patient and check that things are OK. Some pharmacists have arranged for patients to collect their medicines on a weekly basis and have arranged with the GP that weekly prescriptions are provided to enable closer monitoring.

Depression is an area of mental health where patients are known to drop out of treatment with medicines, sometimes before they have had a chance to work. Research indicates that some patients do not receive information (or they receive it but forget it) about how long they can expect to have to take the treatment before they will start to feel better (at least 2 weeks and, more realistically, at least 3–4 weeks). Information about common side-effects is often not discussed with the patient, who may stop taking the treatment as a result of these effects. Tolerance to side-effects can be built up if this is explained to the patient and they are prepared to continue treatment for a while longer. However, an individual patient's response to antidepressants varies, and an assurance needs to be given that if the side-effects continue at the same level and are intolerable, the treatment can be changed. In some areas, antidepressant therapy is dispensed in instalments in the early weeks so that the pharmacist can monitor how the patient is responding to treatment, referring back to the GP where needed.

Pharmacists might consider entering all prescriptions for antidepressants and schizophrenia onto their PMRs, even where the patient is not a regular client of the pharmacy. Such a policy enables the pharmacist to follow up progress with the patient on the next occasion a presciption is presented.

6.7   Osteoporosis and accidents

The treatments to prevent osteoporosis in those at risk now include HRT, alendronate/etidronate and the newer SERMs (selective oestrogen receptor modifiers) such as raloxifene. The potential risks of HRT have been publicized in the media in a manner disproportionate to promotion of benefits. Patients understandably are concerned by reading about the risks of treatment, particularly in relation to breast cancer. The drop-out rate in HRT treatment is high (in some studies only 30 per cent of women continuing with the treatment after 1 year). Possible reasons in addition to concerns about long-term adverse effects include practical effects such as the re-occurrence of bleeds, which some women find unacceptable. Providing the opportunity to discuss these issues at the start of treatment can help women to make an informed choice. For further discussion on these areas, see Chapter 12, Women's health.

These examples illustrate how an awareness of the thoughts and concerns that patients have about medicines can be used to open discussions about treatment. The outcome of pharmacists' interventions may not always be that the patient decides to continue with the treatment. However, better-informed patients who feel that their concerns have been addressed are able to make an informed choice, and the pharmacist's role in concordance is to help them reach that stage.

References

Some of the material in this chapter is based on ideas included in a continuing education module for *Pharmacy Magazine* (A. Blenkinsopp and D. K. Raynor. From compliance to concordance. *Pharmacy Magazine*, 1998)

Britten, N. (1994) Patients ideas about medicines: a qualitative study. *British Journal of General Practice* 44, 465–8.
Coulter, A. (1998) Shared decision-making. *Journal of Health Services Policy and Research*
RPSGB (1997) *From compliance to concordance.* Royal Pharmaceutical Society, London.

7 Smoking

Tobacco is the single most important, avoidable cause of death in developed countries, and an estimated 500 million of the world's current population will die from tobacco-related illness. A further 2.5 million will die prematurely, with an average loss of 20 years of life. In total, this group will lose a total of 5 billion life years. In Britain, more than one in four adults smoke cigarettes. Smoking-related morbidity costs the NHS an estimated £1.7 billion per year. In 1997, the Health Education Authority (HEA) reported that smoking cessation interventions are highly cost-effective in producing population health gains. Pharmacists are ideally placed to give advice and support to smokers about cessation. The White Paper *Smoking Kills* (DH, 1998) recognizes the pharmacist's role in giving smoking cessation advice. Clinical trials throughout the world have shown that nicotine replacement therapy (NRT) doubles the success rate of those attempting to give up when compared with placebo. Most forms of NRT are only available from pharmacies, so pharmacists are in a unique position to support smoking cessation. The government are working closely with the manufacturers of NRT products and with community pharmacists and doctors to improve the provision of on the spot advice and NRT.

7.1 Epidemiology

Smoking is the major cause of morbidity and mortality from cardiovascular disease, chronic respiratory disease, and cancers of the lung and other sites. Smoking is the most important cause of premature death in developed countries and accounts for 120 000 deaths a year in the UK—more than 13 an hour, one-fifth of all deaths. The avoidance of smoking in the UK would eliminate one-third of cancer deaths and one-sixth of deaths from other causes.

A person who smokes regularly more than doubles his or her chances of dying before the age of 65.

In 1974 in Great Britain, 45 per cent of the adult population were smokers, this had reduced to 27 per cent in 1994, but increased to 28 per cent in 1996. The decline has been confined to adults over 35 years. There are large inequalities between socio-economic groups: in the period between 1974 and 1994 smoking prevalence in professional groups fell by half, but in unskilled, manual workers the fall was only a third. So, by 1994, unskilled workers were nearly three times more likely to smoke than professionals. In 1996, 12 per cent of men and 11 per cent of women in the highest socio-economic group smoked. Rates of smoking in the poorest group remain at over 60 per cent. There is evidence that socio-economic status also influences cigarette brand choice and smoking uptake.

The vast majority take up the habit as teenagers. Smoking prevalence in schoolchildren (age 11–15) in 1996 was 15 per cent of girls and 11 per cent of boys. Only 10 per cent of people start smoking after the age of 18, and by the age of 15, 63 per cent of girls and 59 per cent of boys will have tried smoking. One in three 15-year-old girls smoke. An Exeter schools study showed that only 16 per cent of 14- to 15-year-old smokers said they do not want to give up.

The retrospective 1995 Infant Feeding Survey indicated that the percentage of smokers who gave up during pregnancy increased from 24 per cent in 1985 to 33 per cent in 1995. Additionally, 47 per cent smoked fewer cigarettes. The HEA prospective survey, Trends in Smoking and Pregnancy 1992–1997, showed that more than twice as many women with partners in the unemployed and manual groups smoked compared with those with partners in the non-manual group, and only one in four women gave up smoking during pregnancy.

There are estimated to be over a billion smokers in the world, with almost one-third of them living in China. Tobacco consumption has increased in France, Germany, Austria, Denmark, Sweden, Greece, Italy, Spain, Portugal, and Japan, but has decreased in Finland, The Netherlands, Switzerland, Australia, Canada, and North America. There is an increasing prevalence of smoking in developing countries and in Eastern Europe. Many of the world's poorest countries have seen increasing male tobacco consumption and limited regulatory measures. For example, in sub-Saharan Africa, cheap brands have been marketed using intensive advertising, sponsorship of events, and cigarette price wars.

7.1.1 How smoking damages health

The tar content of cigarettes is the single most important factor in terms of health risk. Tar reduction reduces the risk of developing some smoking-related disease, notably lung cancer. However, this is a small reduction and does not compare with the benefit of giving up smoking. Consumers particularly in the higher socio-economic groups are switching to low-tar products; however, smoking of hand-rolled cigarettes that yield more tar because of the use of non-porous paper and the lack of filters, is increasing.

By far the most harmful property of nicotine is its addictiveness. Smokers seek an optimum nicotine dose and, if yields are reduced, will compensate by smoking each cigarette more intensively or by increasing the number of cigarettes they smoke. Nicotine has been shown to have effects on brain dopamine systems similar to those of cocaine and heroin. Dependence is established early on in teenage smoking careers, and adult smoking behaviour is motivated by the need to maintain the addiction. Nicotine withdrawal is incredibly difficult and is an important factor in the failure of many cessation attempts.

Carbon monoxide is produced as a result of the slow combustion process of tobacco smoking. The carbon monoxide yield from cigarettes has decreased over the last 25 years. Carbon monoxide combines irreversibly with haemoglobin to form carboxyhaemoglobin, restricting the uptake and subsequent carriage of oxygen. Research suggests that nitric oxide in tobacco smoke has a detrimental effect on the physiological function of endogenous nitric oxide.

7.2   Health risks from smoking

A large number of fatal and life-threatening diseases are caused by smoking. These include chronic obstructive pulmonary disease, vascular disease, and cancers. Smoking also affects the developing fetus. Environmental tobacco smoke has been linked to sudden infant death, respiratory diseases in childhood, lung cancer, and ischaemic heart disease.

7.2.1 Chronic obstructive pulmonary disease

Chronic bronchitis and emphysema are major causes of death and disability. In a prospective study of British doctors, smokers had 13 times the risk of dying from COPD than non-smokers. Three-quarters of deaths from COPD were attributed to smoking. In addition, cigarette smokers of all ages have more chest disease than non-smokers. In the pharmacy, advice about treatment for coughs is often sought by patients who smoke.

7.2.2 Smoking and vascular disease

Smoking causes extensive arterial damage. Diseases related to smoking include coronary artery disease and heart attacks, aortic aneurysms which can cause sudden death, carotid artery disease which can lead to stroke, and peripheral vascular disease which can lead to severe leg pain when walking and may lead to amputation.

7.2.3 Smoking and cancer

Smoking causes 81 per cent of lung cancers and is also implicated in cancers of the oral cavity, pharynx, larynx, oesophagus, pancreas, and bladder. Many cancers of the mouth and pharynx are caused by a combination of smoking and excessive alcohol intake. Oral cancer can be easily detected, and early treatment is successful.

7.2.4 Smoking in pregnancy

Smoking in pregnancy causes a number of adverse outcomes, including miscarriage, reduced birth weight, and prenatal death. It may also increase the risk of congenital defects such as cleft palate and congenital limb abnormalities. Twenty four per cent of women smoke during pregnancy, and only 33 per cent of women smokers give up during pregnancy. Pharmacists have regular contact with women who are trying to conceive and who are pregnant. These contacts are ideal opportunities to offer support and practical help

on giving up smoking. Research has shown that prenatal counselling lasting up to 10 minutes can double quit rates.

7.2.5 Smoking and tooth loss

Smoking plays a large part in the development of periodontitis, the
major cause of tooth loss, and has been shown to be an independent
risk factor for the development of the disease. Pharmacists can
encourage the public to have regular dental health checks.

Other diseases that may be associated with smoking include
cataracts and hip fractures (osteoporosis).

7.2.6 Smoking and cognitive performance and mood

In habitual smokers, nicotine does not appear to enhance performance. The evidence that smoking relieves stress is weak and the
reverse is true. Contrary to popular belief, stress and anxiety are
decreased after giving up smoking. There is evidence of association
between stress and negative mood states.

7.2.7 Diseases with a lower risk in smokers

There is evidence that smoking reduces the risk of a few diseases
such as Parkinson's disease, ulcerative colitis, and endometrial
cancer; this is probably due to nicotine. Alzheimer's disease is more
complex and it cannot be concluded that smoking reduces the risk
of developing the disease. Research suggests that, overall, smokers
are about four times more likely to develop Alzeimer's disease.
However, there is a subgroup of smokers with a specific genotype
who are less likely than the general population to develop this
disease. It must be emphasized that any benefits conferred by
smoking are far outweighed by the large risks.

7.2.8 Passive smoking

There is increasing evidence that environmental tobacco smoke has
adverse effects on health. There is an increased risk of lung cancer
of the order of 20–30 per cent in those with long-term exposure to
environmental tobacco smoke. Ischaemic heart disease is caused by

environmental tobacco smoke—more research is needed to validate
what is probably a substantial risk. Childhood asthma and other
respiratory illnesses are strongly linked to parental smoking. Parental
smoking is also linked to acute and chronic middle ear disease in
children, and this association is likely to be causal. Sudden infant
death syndrome (cot death) is associated with exposure to tobacco
smoke. Pharmacists can play a very important role in public
education about the risks of smoking in the home in relation to
respiratory disease in children, as well as the risks during pregnancy
and postnatally.

7.3   Influences on tobacco consumption

Four major issues appear to contribute to smoking prevalence:
price, promotion, public education, and social environment.
Cigarette smoking has been shown to decline with regular price
increases above the rate of inflation. Consumption decreases by
around 0.5 per cent for a 1 per cent increase in price; the effect
is greater in lower socio-economic groups. The 1998 report of
the Scientific Committee on Smoking and Health states that the
marketing objectives of the tobacco industry are: to encourage
smokers to consume more cigarettes, to undermine motivation to
quit, to encourage former smokers to begin again, to encourage
adults to start smoking, and to hope that the young will experiment
and therefore become a pool of new customers. It has been
suggested that 300 new smokers are needed per day to replace those
who die from smoking-related diseases.

An estimated £60–100 million was spent on promotion of
tobacco in the UK in 1994 and is described by the industry as
brand strengthening. The tobacco companies fund a body FOREST
(Freedom Organization for the Right to Enjoy Smoking Tobacco)
to counter anti-smoking lobbies such as ASH (Action on Smoking
and Health). Generic promotion is subtle and is carried out by
role models such as television personalities, pop and film stars,
and fashion models. Sports sponsorship serves to promote brands
but also to subvert the argument that smoking is a health risk by
association with healthy sports. The Formula One racing car has
been described as 'the most powerful advertising space in the

world'. A number of countries have banned tobacco advertising, and the European Union recently have signed an agreement to phase it out over the next few years (from 1998). All tobacco sponsorship for global events will be ended by 2006. Tobacco advertising bans in Norway and Finland reduced consumption by 9 and 7 per cent, respectively. Bans in Canada, Australia, and New Zealand led to smaller reductions. The White Paper *Smoking Kills* states that the UK government will end tobacco advertising on billboards and printed media by the end of 1999.

The government have committed £50 million over the next 3 years (from 1999) to develop a sustained and coordinated health education campaign. The campaign will focus on teenagers, less well off adults, pregnant women, and mothers. The government will explore the scope for collaborative work with pharmacy.

Extensive health education campaigns by government bodies such as the HEA and by pressure groups such as ASH have publicized the health risks of smoking to a large audience. Social pressures to stop smoking are growing, particularly in the professional groups. Most public transport, parts of many cinemas and theatres, many shops, and most work places have banned smoking. Many restaurants, cafes, and a small number of pubs have banned smoking or provide non-smoking areas. Many airlines have banned smoking on all flights, although these airlines still sell duty-free cigarettes on their flights. Charter air companies have still to be convinced of the benefits of banning smoking on flights. North America is way ahead of other countries on this, and smoking in public is increasingly taboo.

7.4   Smoking cessation

Government targets—the government have set smoking cessation targets for England and there are also targets for Scotland, Wales, and Northern Ireland.

Children—aim: to stop the rise in children smoking

target: to reduce smoking among children from 13 to 9 per cent or less by the year 2010; with a fall to 11 per cent by the year 2005. This will mean approximately 110 000 fewer children smoking in England by the year 2010.

Adults—aim: to establish a new downward trend in adult smoking rates in all social classes

target: to reduce adult smoking in all social classes so that the overall rate falls from 28 per cent to 24 per cent or less by the year 2010; with a fall to 26 per cent by the year 2005. In terms of today's population, this would mean 1.5 million fewer smokers in England.

Smoking during pregnancy—aim: to improve the health of expectant mothers and their families

target: to reduce the percentage of women who smoke during pregnancy from 23 per cent to 15 per cent by the year 2010; with a fall to 18 per cent by the year 2005. This will mean approximately 55 000 fewer women in England who smoke during pregnancy.

7.4.1 Interventions by health professionals

The conclusions of two major systematic reviews and an HEA cost-effectiveness review are that people will stop smoking as a result of brief, unsolicited advice from health professionals. There is strong research evidence for the effectiveness of brief (less than 3 minutes) opportunistic advice compared with none; 3–10 minutes counselling is even more effective. If follow up is provided, this enhances the chances of quitting in motivated individuals. The only strategy that has been shown convincingly to enhance the effectiveness of professional advice is provision of NRT; it appears to double the odds of quitting and this is an effect largely independent of the amount of advice provided. There have been calls for work to develop strategies to increase the frequency with which smokers are identified and offered advice and support.

Prochaska, DiClemente and colleagues have pioneered and widely researched the transtheoretical model (see Chapter 4) to explain how people intentionally modify addictive behaviour such as smoking. The model involves a cyclical pattern of movement through specific stages of change and a common set of processes of change that seem to be independent of demographics and problem history. They have determined that efficient self-change depends on doing the right things at the right time (stages).

For smoking the stages are:

Pre-contemplation—smokers are not thinking about quitting, at least not in the next 6 months.

Contemplation—the period of time in which smokers are seriously considering quitting smoking during the next 6 months

Preparation—the period in which smokers are seriously thinking about quitting smoking in the next month

Action—the period ranging from 0 to 6 months when smokers have made the overt change to stop smoking

Maintenance—the period beginning 6 months after the action stage has started and continuing until smoking is terminated as a problem.

Studies have shown that the vast majority of smokers are not prepared to take action for their smoking, yet most health promotion programmes have been designed for the small minority of smokers who are prepared for action. Prochaska and colleagues designed interventions for the majority of smokers who are in the pre-contemplation and contemplation stages of change. Their programmes are designed to help smokers learn from their quit attempts, rather than become demoralized by their failures. They have used interactive multimedia computers successfully to give patients tailored feedback about their smoking and what they could change in order to become non-smokers.

In a Cochrane review, health care professionals who had received training were significantly more likely to perform tasks relating to smoking cessation than untrained controls. The effects of training were enhanced if prompts and reminders were sent to the health care professionals to reinforce the training messages. The review stated that organizational factors are important to ensure that smoking cessation measures are delivered reliably. Training, said the review, is expensive, and providing training without addressing the constraints imposed by the conditions in which health professionals practice is unlikely to be a wise use of resources. The authors call for studies about training health care professionals other than doctors, and say that pharmacists as well as nurses and physiotherapists are well placed to facilitate smoking cessation.

In a robust study involving pharmacist training in the Grampian Region of Scotland, a 2-hour training package based on the HEA's Stages of Change model of smoking cessation was used to train pharmacists and counter assistants. Participants felt that the model was a good way of understanding smoking cessation, and reported that the training was a good learning experience; they had been able to utilize the training, it had made a difference to the way they counselled customers, and had increased job satisfaction. Those patients who were counselled by the participants were significantly more likely than those who used the control pharmacies to be not smoking when followed up.

A recent analysis of the effectiveness of interventions intended to help people stop smoking concluded that non-specific behaviour modification in the form of relaxation, rewards and punishments, and avoiding trigger situations do not have a significant effect on cessation. Contrary to popular perceptions, sudden cessation and gradual cessation are on average similar in their efficacy. The effects of using nurses in health promotion clinics and other treatments, such as clonidine, aversion therapy, and hypnosis, are unclear. Supportive group sessions, aversion with silver acetate gum or spray, sensory deprivation, tranquillisers, and acupuncture were all ineffective.

7.4.2   Nicotine replacement therapy

Simple advice to quit, that will probably only take a couple of minutes, backed up by ongoing support (i.e. asking the client how they are getting on each time they come in to the pharmacy) and supplying NRT for highly dependent smokers (more than 15 cigarettes per day) is the most effective way to help smokers to quit. All pharmacists and counter assistants can provide this level of service within the constraints of current practice.

A recent Cochrane review determined the effectiveness of different forms of NRT in achieving abstinence from cigarettes. It involved 23 700 smokers in 47 trials of nicotine gum, 22 of transdermal nicotine patches, three of intranasal spray, and two of inhaled nicotine. The authors concluded that offering any form of NRT is better than nothing or placebo. It is not possible to compare treatments directly because the trials are for individual products versus placebo and not versus each other. The two factors which seem to be the major determinants of the effectiveness of NRT are the setting in which it is offered and the smoker's level of dependence upon nicotine. These two factors are far greater than the nature and flexibility of the dosage regimen. Cessation using

NRT is likely to be achieved sooner than if several unsupported and likely-to-fail attempts are made. This results in life years gained by the use of NRT being nearly three times as many as those gained by brief counselling.

It must be remembered that many of the trials have been conducted with community volunteers or those attending specialized clinics (who may be more motivated to quit) rather than in more pragmatic settings such as community pharmacies. The authors caution about being influenced by advertisements into thinking that NRT is a miracle cure. They state that quitting smoking is not a one-off event and that many smokers only give up after several attempts. They say that falsely raising the expectations of smokers who purchase over-the-counter NRT, via advertising, without at least providing minimal support and an adequate explanation of the limitations of using NRT, may be counterproductive. This serves to endorse the role of pharmacists. They conclude that all the commercially available forms of NRT are effective as part of a strategy to promote smoking cessation. NRT, they say, should be directed to smokers who are motivated to quit and have high levels of nicotine dependence. They call for further comparisons of available forms of NRT. It would be prudent to carry out at least some of these trials in a community pharmacy setting where most NRT is supplied.

Myths surrounding nicotine replacement therapy

There are several misconceptions about nicotine and NRT, the most important being the possibility that nicotine is damaging to health and the potential for a person to become addicted to NRT. There is no evidence that nicotine is carcinogenic. The dose of nicotine delivered by NRT is much lower than that in cigarettes and dependence is not a significant problem. The WHO have concluded that there is not significant abuse of NRT and that there is no need to review this aspect. Adverse effects from NRT are rare, usually slight, and of limited duration. Research has demonstrated the safety of NRT in patients with existing heart disease, although product licences still preclude its over-the-counter use in such patients.

NRT can alleviate many of the objective and subjective effects of stopping smoking such as gastrointestinal disturbances, sleep problems, irritability, and the loss of concentration and memory. Two recent reports, *Standing Committee On Tobacco and Health* and *A call for a more effective UK public policy on smoking cessation and the use of NRT* have called for NRT to be more widely available. Availability of NRT on NHS prescription would have short-term financial implications for the health service's drugs bill although the long-term financial benefits could potentially be great through a substantial reduction in smoking-related morbidity. If NRT was available on prescription, it could help health care professionals to target the poorer people in society. If NRT could be prescribed in hospital, it could help the many people who attempt to quit following admission for smoking-related conditions.

7.4.3 Facts about the benefits of giving up

- In 20 minutes, blood pressure and pulse rate return to normal
- *In 8 hours, CO levels reduce by half and oxygen levels return to normal*
- After:
  1 day, lungs start to clear of mucus
  2 days, the senses of taste and smell improve
  3 days, breathing becomes easier and bronchioles begin to relax
  2–12 weeks, circulation improves
  3–9 months, lung function increases by up to 10 per cent
  5 years, the risk of heart attack falls to half that of a smoker
  10 years, the risk of lung cancer falls to half that of a smoker
  10 years, the risk of heart attack falls to the same as someone who never smoked.

Physiological effects of giving up

Explaining the physiological effects of quitting can prepare people about what to expect.

- Cough may initially worsen as ciliary clearance begins
- Some people feel light headed or dizzy as the oxygen supply to the brain increases
- Improved peripheral circulation may cause tingling in the hands and feet

- Diarrhoea or constipation may occur
- Mood swings and irritability are common.

7.4.4 Pharmacy-based smoking cessation services

Pharmacists can offer a smoking cessation service using the Stages of Change model. Pharmacists and their staff can both respond to requests from people who want to quit and offer opportunistic advice. The use of the model in the pharmacy setting offers these benefits:

- Helping to move smokers from the contemplation and preparation stages to the action and maintenance stages where the use of NRT is appropriate
- Improving the effectiveness of NRT by reducing its inappropriate use through targeting at smokers at the correct stages of the model
- Increasing the chance of smoking cessation success by providing important additional support matched to the need of the individual
- Being more effective in terms of use of pharmacists' and assistants' time by reducing inappropriate intervention
  (From Sinclair *et al.*, 1997)

Pharmacists need to practice questioning techniques that will help them to assess which stage the individual is at. Questions should aim to get the person to talk about their current thoughts, and examples would include:

- Have you ever thought about stopping?
- Would you like some information about stopping?
- Do you think you are ready to try to stop?
- Would you like to try to stop?
- Do you think nicotine replacement therapy might help you to stop?

The answers will help the pharmacist to assess what response would be appropriate. The key point is not to try to push the person to move from one stage to the next, but to provide information, support, and treatment where the person's responses suggest these are needed.

A number of innovative pharmacists run smoking cessation clinics. Individuals who participate are encouraged to visit the pharmacy regularly for follow up and support. In Northern Ireland, Terry Maguire developed the PAS (Pharmacists Action on Smoking) model, later adopted by many community pharmacists who joined the PAS group. The PAS system involves pharmacist and NRT support for people who are ready to stop smoking. It has been evaluated recently using clinical trial methodology, a 14 per cent 1 year cessation rate was shown, compared with 2 per cent for controls.

7.5   Case studies

1. You are talking with a man aged 35 who has asthma and recently started to bring his prescriptions to your pharmacy. You ask if he smokes. He does. You ask if he has thought about stopping. He says he is not interested and is sick of his doctor, who tells him to stop every time he sees him. A few months later, he says he has been thinking and would like to try to stop. You discuss this with him and advise him appropriately. A few weeks later, he comes in and says he has started again.

In the initial conversation, this man was at the pre-contemplation stage and would have been unreceptive to approaches from the pharmacist. However, several months later, he has moved through the contemplation stage and goes on to try to quit. There may be a long lag time between pre-contemplation and contemplation. The pharmacist can check out from time to time whether the person has moved from their last stage. Relapse is common, and many smokers take several attempts to quit. This is part of the cyclical nature of the Stages of Change model. The pharmacist can reassure him and find out what stage of the cycle he is at, and whether he is ready for another attempt to quit now.

2. A young woman aged about 20 has come into the pharmacy and asked you to do a pregnancy test.

The result is positive, and the woman is delighted. You ask if she has been taking folic acid and, on finding that she has not, recommend that she takes it until week 12 of her pregnancy. You ask if she smokes and explain that many women do try to stop smoking when they fall pregnant because of the effect on the developing fetus and on young childrens' health. She tells you that her friend told her that you have a smaller baby if you smoke, which makes the birth easier. Besides, she will put on weight too and she does not want to do that. She also says that smoking is one of her few pleasures in life and that her boyfriend smokes too, so unless he gave up it would be impossible.

This woman is in the 'pre-contemplation' stage of the Prochaska and diClemente model and is not thinking about giving up. The pharmacist can provide information and support here. The pharmacist must realize that the woman feels defensive about her smoking and try to show her that she is concerned about her health and the health of the unborn baby. She can provide the woman with information about the benefits of stopping smoking during pregnancy which far outweigh having a small baby, and the benefits of continuing not to smoke after the birth. Although many women give up for the duration of the pregnancy, many resume smoking after their child is born. The pharmacist can ask the woman how many cigarettes she smokes a day and suggest that she could use the money saved to buy things for the baby. If the woman smoked 20 cigarettes a day at £3.50 per pack, she would save over £1200 in a year to spend on the baby. The pharmacist can also address the problem of weight gain during pregnancy, telling the woman it is normal to put on weight during pregnancy. The pharmacist can emphasize that putting on a few pounds is much less harmful to health than continuing to smoke, and that the weight can be lost through healthy eating and exercise both during the pregnancy and after the baby is born. The pharmacist can encourage the woman to at least try to cut down on the amount of cigarettes that she is smoking. The pharmacist can provide the woman with written information and invite her to come back if she wants to discuss it further.

3. A man in his thirties comes in to the pharmacy and asks for some patches to help him give up smoking. He tells the pharmacist that he smokes at least a packet of cigarettes a day.

This man is in the 'preparation' stage, and seems to be ready to enter the 'action' stage; he has decided to stop and wants some help to do so. He tells you he has tried to stop before but gets too irritable and always starts again; he has heard that the patches will help him to wean off smoking without feeling so bad. The pharmacist should offer the man encouragement and tell him that the nicotine patches will certainly help him to avoid some of the effects of giving up smoking. The pharmacist should then check if the man has any serious diseases such as heart disease, a recent stroke, diabetes, generalized skin disease, liver or kidney disease, stomach ulcer, or overactive thyroid. In patients with concurrent diseases, patches will still be useful and it must be remembered that the nicotine delivered by transdermal patches is of a much smaller dose than that from cigarettes so will cause fewer cardiovascular and endocrine side-effects. If the pharmacist is in any doubt about recommending NRT to a particular person, they should discuss it with the person's GP.

The pharmacist should encourage the man to think about the situations when he will miss smoking the most, for example at coffee breaks, in the pub, after a meal, and should suggest appropriate behavioural changes, for example to do something else to occupy himself straight after a meal, to go to a different place for his coffee break, or to avoid the pub for a couple of weeks.

The pharmacist should also give advice about applying and using the patches. The manufacturers provide material to back up the use of all NRT products, and the pharmacist should be familiar with the advice for each product. The pharmacist should encourage the man to come back and tell them how he is getting on when he purchases more patches and to contact them if he needs further support. When he does return to the pharmacy, the pharmacist should make sure that the assistants know that they should encourage him and ask him how he is getting on.

4. *A middle aged man, who works in the local factory, is a regular visitor to the pharmacy in the winter months for cough mixtures.*

The pharmacist has trained the assistants to ask the WHAM questions to everyone who asks for a medicine, who is the medicine for?, what are the symptoms?, how long have they been present, any action taken? (particularly medicines tried already), and what regular medicines are being taken? However, this questioning sequence is unlikely to reveal whether or not a person is a smoker. Since more than one in four people smoke, it would not be unreasonable to include a question about smoking in the questioning sequence. If the man was a smoker, the assistants could be trained to ask if he had ever considered stopping smoking and to tell him that the pharmacy can offer advice and support to help people who want to stop. The man may be aware that smoking is causing his chronic chest complaint and may be at the contemplation stage and value some advice.

References

Department of Health (1998) *Smoking kills*. The Stationery Office, London.

Sinclair, H. K., Bond. C. M., Lennox, A. S., Winfield, A. J. and Taylor, R. J. (1995) Nicotine replacement therapies: smoking cessation outcomes in a pharmacy setting in Scotland. *Tobacco Control* 4, 338–43.

Sinclair, H. K., Bond, C., Lennox, A. S., Silcock, J., and Winfield, A. (1997) An evaluation of a training workshop for pharmacists based on the Stages of Change model of smoking cessation. *Health Education Journal* 56, 296–312.

8 Nutrition

From the 1930s onwards, thinking and education on nutrition was based on the premise that the population should receive a balanced diet—that is, to prevent malnourishment. This was of great importance at a time of widespread economic deprivation and ensured that people received sufficient amounts of protein, carbohydrate, minerals, and essential fats.

During the 1950s and 1960s, a more affluent society became aware of the need to prevent becoming overweight, and there developed a commonly held belief that some foods, such as cheese, were essentially 'good', and others were equally 'bad', and here all carbohydrates were grouped together including potatoes and bread.

Two major factors began to change this view in the 1970s—the rising death toll from coronary heart disease and the awareness that this was linked to nutrition, and to the rising amount of processed food in the diet. Researchers began to compare the morbidity rates with those during and after the war where the population, on a very restricted diet which was low in fat and processed food, was healthier than that 20 years later. Research evidence now shows that diet is linked to many diseases and symptoms.

In the 1990s, the poorest are worse off—in absolute terms, that is adjusting for inflation—than they were in 1979. One-quarter of the adult population have no significant assets, and it is estimated that one-quarter of children live in poverty. Even if the poorest had stayed ahead of inflation, they would have fallen further behind the rest of us, resulting in loneliness, exclusion, and the inability to do the rest of the things we take for granted. As Sir Donald Acheson said in a speech on his report on poverty and health (1998)

'Poverty is not just of matter of money. It is a question of how far you have to walk, with a pushchair, in the rain, to a shop that sells food that you can afford to spend it on'.

8.1   Diet and disease

Research evidence has now shown that there are strong relationships between diet and ill- health.

The link between diet and disease

- Cardiovascular conditions
  Coronary heart disease
  Hypertension
  Stroke
- Gastrointestinal tract
  Indigestion
  Heartburn
  Constipation
  Irritable bowel syndrome
  Diverticulosis
- Cancers
  Nearly one-third have been linked to diet
- Allergy
  Coeliac disease
  Lactose intolerance
  Eczema
  Hayfever
  Migraine
- Others
  Vitamin deficiencies
  Eating disorders

Mounting concern about diet and health led to the setting up of special committees and the publication of two key reports in the 1980s which summarized current research on nutrition and disease. Although it is now over a decade since they first appeared, their main messages remain relevant today. The NACNE (National Advisory Committee on Nutrition Education) report published in 1983 examined the British diet in relation to a wide range of conditions. The following year, the COMA (Committee on Medical Aspects of Food Policy) report *Diet and cardiovascular disease* (1984) was published, setting out how diet should be changed to prevent heart disease. The two reports were in broad agreement that the amount of total energy derived from dietary fat should be reduced, that there should be a reduction in the intake of saturated fat, and that there was some evidence to support a small increase in the intake of polyunsaturated fats.

In 1988, the WHO published a report with recommendations for healthy eating in Europe, *Nutrition and health*, which proposed reductions in fats, sugar, and salt and an increase in dietary fibre. COMA published a second report *Dietary sugars and human disease* in 1989. Two further COMA reports were published on cardio-vascular disease in 1994 and on nutritional aspects of the development of cancer in 1998. The World Cancer Research Fund published a report in 1997 which estimated that 30–40 percent of cancers are preventable if an appropriate diet is eaten. There has also been much developmental work on the dietary reference values of food energy—published in a Department of Health report (*Dietary reference values for food energy and nutrients in the UK*, 1991, Report no. 41).

8.1.1   Nutrition: the consumer's agenda

Since the key reports were published, there has been an increase in public awareness not only about healthier eating but also about concern at the way animals and reared and managed. Public outcry at the way calves were tethered and the way pigs were bred, as well as factory farming of chickens, has resulted in legislation to change some of these practices and change patterns of consumption. The dangers of the use of pesticides have also been publicized and have encouraged the organic farming of vegetables and other foods. While the cost remains higher, the uptake will remain small. There is no nutritional difference between organically produced food and the standard produce.

The saga of bovine spongiform encephalopathy (BSE) and the mixed messages given by government spokesmen more concerned with protecting the farming lobby than truly informing consumers resulted in British beef being banned by the EC and clear evidence of the disease crossing the species barrier. Lack of information has made the problem worse—a salutary lesson for the future. This is shown by the current debate on genetically modified foods and their

production, which has demonstrated that the public's belief that
governments are to be trusted without question has disappeared
forever.

It is of increasing importance that we have started the global
debate of the extent to which the planet will be damaged if we
continue to condone the destruction of rain forests and the huge use
of energy in continuing to offer the western world a meat-rich diet.

There is also greater awareness of eating disorders, with many
highly publicized cases of prominent people with anorexia and
bulimia. Here too, there is rising consumer awareness of the media's
role in promoting the concept that to be underweight is to be
beautiful. Complaints to fashion magazines using clearly anorexic
models have made them aware of the strength of public feeling.

This rise in awareness—of how animals are treated, how land is
farmed, and of the power of the media in portraying an image of
beauty that promotes ill-health—reinforces the message of the first
chapters in this book, that is that health is perceived differently by
different people and a holistic approach will indeed consider not
just the fat content, but how the food was brought to the table.
Many of the changes needed for a healthy and renewable diet need
legislation at the national or international level as well as a change
in funding welfare to ensure that children in deprived families
receive an adequate diet.

What of the pharmacist's role in all this? As we have already said,
there is the now recognized role of all health professionals in
promoting health, and pharmacists are very much part of this. So
this chapter focuses on the key health messages—reduce total fat,
eat more fruit and vegetables, reduce sugar and salt, and increase
fibre. Pharmacists are asked many more questions on nutrition and
it is not the scope of this book to address all of these, but certainly
to recognize the value of the role. People can often be confused by
what appear to be (or are) contradictory reports and scares about
what we eat and drink, and the pharmacy is a source of unbiased
and good advice.

The specialist reports referred to above make the same recommendations. These are that the amount of sugar in the diet should
be reduced and that less salt should be eaten. The amount of fibre in
the diet should be increased. They note with concern the rise in
consumption of dairy foods and that sugar is added to many foods.

The consumer has little idea that this is the case or indeed of the percentage.

Fibre is removed from many foods during processing, and there is widespread public belief that eating carbohydrates (and fibre is contained in many carbohydrates such as pulses) is likely to result in weight gain. In the public's mind, therefore, carbohydrates are 'fattening' and should be avoided. In fact, excess calories and consequent weight gain are more likely to be found in saturated fats and sugar consumed or in the way in which carbohydrates are being cooked—the British diet of 'chips with everything'.

The main dietary recommendations are as follows.

Fat intake

The percentage of total energy derived from fat should be reduced for most people. Much of this reduction can be achieved by eating fewer dairy foods, for example by changing from full-fat to semi-skimmed milk, by eating low-fat spreads, and by reducing the amount of hard cheese. Reducing the amount of red meat and changing to white meat such as chicken is another recommended way of achieving this goal.

Fats are solid at room temperature, while oils, made from pressed olives for example, are liquid. Both are fatty acids, but they behave differently—the 'essential' fatty acids, which we need, are poly-unsaturates made by plants. They come in two main forms—linoleic (the *n*6 family where the *n* refers to the position of the double bond nearest the non-oxygen end of the molecule) and linolenic acid (the *n*3 family). The *n*6 family predominates in most green plants, although some plants in hotter climates store energy as saturated fat—examples being avocado and coconut. Sheep and cows eat unsaturated fats and convert them into saturated ones, but fish do not do this. Hence fish are rich in unsaturated fatty acids of the *n*3 series, and the oily fish—mackerel, herring, sardines, and pilchards—have the acids in their muscles, that is the part we eat.

Changing the method of cooking from frying to grilling or baking, or using low-fat oils for frying are effective ways to reduce fat intake. COMA recommended 35 per cent and the WHO report 30 per cent of total energy as fat. One change, for example from full-fat to semi-skimmed milk, would go halfway towards this goal.

Sugar

Again, we should eat as little as possible and be aware of the sugar content of processed foods by reading the labels. Many consumers might expect sweet things to contain sugar but would be surprised to know that powdered soups, baked beans, and muesli also contain sugar. Another source of surprise at the time of the first reports was the sheer volume of sugar in products such as yoghurt. Sugar-free and reduced sugar products are now on sale, but many other products remain high in sugar.

Salt

The COMA committee's latest recommendation is that everyone should eat no more than 6 g of salt a day. Around 80 per cent of the salt we eat is hidden in processed food, but suggested steps to reduce intake are to discontinue the habit of routinely adding salt when cooking and considering again whether to make it routinely available at the table. Better consumer awareness is needed of the large quantities of salt in some foods, which should be clearly labelled with the salt content.

Cereals, fruit, and vegetables

We should eat more of all of these. They are full of starchy carbohydrate, vitamins, and fibre. Good and cheap products rich in fibre are wholemeal bread, unpeeled potatoes, pulses, and root vegetables. There is a widespread and misconceived belief that to eat more fibre means to eat more salad. Most salad vegetables contain little fibre. Fibre is now known as non-starch polysaccharide (NSP), and later work has clarified the differences between types. It comes in two types—soluble and non-soluble—the former existing in pulses, fruit, and vegetables. Insoluble NSP is in whole wheat cereals and is also sold as processed bran, that is extracted from the cereal.

An American trial in 1997 specifically tested the effect of a diet rich in fruit, vegetables, and low fat dairy products and with reduced saturated and total fat. Results showed a substantial reduction in blood pressure—a major predisposing factor in coronary heart disease.

More recent work has also looked more closely at individual fruits and vegetables, and has found the latter as a class to be more protective against cancers: the cruciferous family (cabbages, broccoli, brussels sprouts, and cauliflower) as well as onions and garlic seem to be of special value.

Antioxidants are also under review, with the underlying hypothesis that it may be their presence in fruit and vegetables which gives the protective effect. To date, trials including antioxidants as supplements have produced ambiguous results.

Alcohol is associated with an increased incidence of cancers of the mouth. The government guidelines are 3 units a day for women and 4 for men. However, the good news for moderate drinkers is that there is reasonable evidence that moderate intake reduces the risk of heart disease

8.2 Health risks

8.2.1 The case for reducing fat in the diet

The major health risk is of coronary heart disease. The higher the cholesterol level in the blood, the greater the risk of heart disease. This risk is proportional to the extent to which the cholesterol level is raised (the 20 per cent of people with the nation's highest cholesterol levels are three times more likely to die of heart disease than the 20 per cent with the lowest levels). When blood cholesterol levels are reduced, either by drugs or by diet, there is an equivalent reduction in the risk of heart disease. High cholesterol levels have been shown in large studies to be one of the three major modifiable risk factors for coronary heart disease (the other two being smoking and hypertension).

A diet which is high in fat is also likely to be high in calories and to lead to weight gain. Thus, dietary fats contribute to the development of overweight and obesity, a further risk factor for heart disease.

The percentage of cholesterol in the blood which is derived from the cholesterol in our diet (from high-cholesterol foods such as egg yolk) is low. Cholesterol is produced by the liver in direct proportion to the amount of saturated fat that is eaten. A common misunderstanding among the public is that only foods which are high in cholesterol are 'bad'. There is a strong case for educating the whole population to more healthy eating patterns, as well as concentrating on those who have high cholesterol levels.

Bowel cancer appears to be linked to a diet which is high in fat and red meat. Research has been unable to identify the relative contribution of two factors, fat and fibre, to the development of bowel cancer.

8.2.2   The case for reducing salt

Salt intake appears to be one of the factors which affect blood pressure, and high blood pressure is a major contributory factor to heart disease and stroke. The incidence of stroke has been reduced over the last 10 years, largely due to the intervention of screening for hypertension and subsequent action either by drug therapy or changes such as weight reduction and reduced salt intake. While the WHO, NACNE, and COMA reports were agreed that salt intake in the UK is too high and that salt appears to play an important part in the development of hypertension, the evidence is not clear-cut.

Research has clearly shown that, in societies where salt intake is low, blood pressure does not rise with age, as is the case in the developed world. In those societies, the incidence of coronary heart disease and stroke is significantly lower. However, it has yet to be proved that a reduction in salt intake in individual diets in the UK has resulted in a proportional reduction in the incidence of hypertension. Population studies are fraught with difficulties—they must be longitudinal (i.e. conducted over many years), take into account other changes in diet and lifestyle, and then demonstrate that one factor has affected the whole. Nonetheless, expert opinion is agreed that a reduction in salt in the diet is likely to be of benefit even though the case for it is not fully proven.

8.2.3   The case for reducing sugar

The most recent survey in the UK showed 43 per cent of males and 29 per cent of females to be overweight, with 13 per cent of men and

16 per cent of women classified as obese The percentage of the population who are obese has been increasing in the UK over a period of several decades. The process begins early in life; by the age of 11 years, 6 per cent of boys and 10 per cent of girls are overweight.

The major dietary contributory factors to weight gain are fats and sugar. At the time that the NACNE report was published, the average sugar consumption in the UK was 38 kg per person annually—double the recommended level. Nutritionists are agreed that sugar is not an essential component of our diet; in fact sugar has been said to provide 'empty calories', that is it has no nutritional value. There is increasing awareness that non-insulin-dependent diabetes is associated with obesity, although no direct causal role for excess sugar intake has been established.

Sugar is implicated in the onset of dental caries. The concern is that young children are most seriously at risk from dental caries, and it is they who are most likely to receive the heavily sugared products, such as fizzy drinks and sweets, which are liable to cause their teeth to rot. Criticism has been levelled at food manufacturers for not clearly stating sugar content, particularly in foods and drinks for babies.

8.2.4   The case for more fibre

All major reports on nutrition recommended an increase in dietary fibre as one of the measures to be taken in reducing the likelihood of coronary heart disease. In this case, the amount of fibre consumed affects the cholesterol level. Research suggests that this is due at least in part to an indirect effect—a reduction in the amount of saturated fats consumed when an individual increases the amount of fibre eaten. However, soluble fibre (found in oats, fruit, vegetables, and pulses) appears to have the effect of reducing cholesterol levels.

The second cause of concern as a result of our low-fibre diet is the incidence of bowel cancer, which is low in countries where fibre intake is high. However, a major study published in 1999 found no association between fibre intake and the incidence of bowel cancer. It is worth noting that low-fibre diets also tend to be high in fats.

The beneficial affect of increased fibre intake on the incidence of constipation is well established. Constipation can range from being merely a troublesome symptom to having much more serious implications—such as the retention of potential toxins and carcinogens in the dietary tract for days rather than hours (thought to increase cancer risk) and the likelihood of developing related conditions, such as diverticular disease or haemorrhoids.

Other conditions which are linked to a low dietary fibre intake are diverticulosis and the irritable bowel syndrome. Patients suffering from either of these are likely to benefit from increasing their intake of fibre.

8.3   Dietary advice from the pharmacist

Eating is, for most people, doing far more than simply keeping malnutrition at bay. This is true even in primitive societies, where the tribe will gather together to share a meal. Food is associated with early childhood memories and pleasures, and what was offered as a treat in childhood is likely to remain so throughout life— witness expensive London restaurants offering food such as bread-and-butter pudding and steamed treacle sponge, remembered presumably from happy schooldays and still much sought-after by middle-aged men.

So it is important to realize that many people cannot change their eating habits easily—if this were not the case, the population would not have such a high percentage of overweight men and women. The behaviour change sought, therefore, which is most likely to succeed, is not to eschew favoured foods totally but to 'ration' them and to substitute others which may become desired in their own right. Thus, if chips, beer, or cream cakes are seen to be desirable foods, then it is pointless to suggest that they be abandoned but, rather, that they should be eaten for 'treats' on special occasions.

The following tables (Tables 8.1–8.4) show the foods that have the greatest percentage of fat, sugar, and salt, and the lowest percentage of fibre, together with the substitutes that can be offered.

Table 8.1 Fat content of foods

High	Low
All fried food, sausages, pate, dairy foods (butter, cream, hard cheeses, full-fat milk), red meat (except lean cuts), mayonnaise, salad cream, suet, potato crisps, meat pies and pasties, margarine	Semi-skimmed and skimmed milk, cottage cheese, low-fat yoghurt, grilled fish, white meat (turkey, chicken, rabbit), all vegetables, potatoes (other than fried), cereals, low-fat cheese, low-fat spreads

Table 8.2 Foods with a high sugar content

Food	Sugar content
Soft drinks	4–8 teaspoonfuls per glass
Desserts	
Ice cream (family block)	9 teaspoonfuls of sugar
Jelly (one packet)	19 teaspoonfuls of sugar
Fruit yoghurt (one carton)	4 teaspoonfuls of sugar
Tinned fruit (one small tin)	5 teaspoonfuls of sugar
Cereals (where sugar is included)	1–2 teaspoonful per serving
Biscuits	one biscuit = 1–2 teaspoonfuls of sugar
Cakes	one slice = 1–4 teaspoonfuls of sugar
Sweet sauces, custard	one serving = 1 teaspoonful of sugar
Soups (tinned/packet)	one bowl = 1–2 teaspoonfuls of sugar
Tinned vegetables	small tin = 1–2 teaspoonfuls of sugar
Confectionery	All confectionery is likely to comprise > 50% sugar

Table 8.3 High-salt foods

Salted peanuts, peanut butter, crisps, yeast extracts

Hard cheeses, bacon, processed meat, sausages, pork/beef pies, smoked fish

Some breakfast cereals (All Bran, Cornflakes), tinned and packet soups, tinned and packet vegetables

Table 8.4   Fibre content of foods

High	Low
Pulses—peas, lentils, etc., wholemeal bread, dried fruit, baked beans, bananas, oranges, brown rice, wholewheat pasta, potatoes in their skins, root vegetables, most leaf vegetables, nuts	Lettuce, cucumber, tomato, white bread, white rice, white pasta

8.4   Over-the-counter and prescription products

8.4.1   For weight loss

Pharmacists are regularly asked to advise about the best product for losing weight quickly, and 'slimming' products are also widely available from other outlets. What is the best advice? Micro diets are also known as VLCD (very low calorie diets) and have an intake of as little as 600 calories per day. Many such products are in the form of a soup or sweet drink mixture, based on skimmed milk, with added vitamins and other nutrients. Such products will, because of their low calorific intake, lead to weight loss, but there are several concerns about their use.

For the people who are overweight and where there is no underlying health disorder, short-term use of a VLCD of up to 4 weeks should pose no risk. However, the long-term effects of a continued calorie intake which is very low are less clear, and the loss of lean tissue in addition to fat can lead to problems. VLCDs have received much publicity and, therefore, close attention, since in the past they have occasioned fatalities. In each case, the women had adhered rigidly to the diet for far longer than the manufacturer's recommendation and the muscle loss was sufficiently great to weaken vital heart muscle. Products now available have manufacturers' instructions which refer to short periods of use. Some people should not use VLCDs at all—these include pregnant women, diabetics, those with heart disease, and children.

However, the major drawback of very low-calorie diets is that healthier eating patterns are not learned. When the diet is stopped, research shows that the majority of people regain their lost weight and even increase from their starting weight. Nonetheless, for some

people, such diets give an encouraging start to weight reduction—
for many people a healthy target.

When pharmacists sell these products, the added instruction should
be given that they should not be taken for more than 4 weeks and
only after having ensured that it is safe for that particular customer
to do so. At the same time, advice can be offered on ways of achieving
weight loss that is likely to be maintained. An agreed change in diet
between the pharmacist and the customer is more likely to have
long-term results. One helpful measure is to ask the customer to
keep a diary of everything they eat during the course of a week. It is
then easy to identify the parts of the diet which are likely to be
causing an increase in weight for reasons of which the customer
may be unaware. Group support has been shown to be an effective
way of maintaining weight loss, and the Weight Watchers organization is one of the few slimming aids found to be effective. Referral
to a dietitian, who may have sessions at the local health centre, for
further advice and counselling is another option. Pharmacists could
contact their local dietitians to establish working links.

Other proprietary products sold to help those wishing to lose
weight are designed as meal substitutes of known and low calorie
content, or to prevent hunger pangs by their fibre content. Good
advice from the pharmacist about high-fibre foods which can
achieve the same effect can be helpful. The fibre content of many
slimming products such as bran tablets is relatively low, and
increasing dietary fibre in other ways is a healthier alternative. The
'natural' snack bars containing dried fruit, bran, and oats are often
high in sugar and are not a low-calorie alternative to sweets

Sweeteners can be a great help for those with 'a sweet tooth'.
In addition to sweetening tablets for hot drinks, granulated forms
are now available which taste virtually the same as sugar. Soft
drinks and dessert products are only two of a wide range of artifi-
cially sweetened foods. While the ideal is to reduce or cut out sugar
completely, such products can be helpful for those who find it
difficult to give up sweet-tasting foods from their diet.

8.4.2 Laxatives

Many pharmacy customers ask for treatment for constipation and,
since a common cause of constipation is insufficient fibre and fluids

in the diet, advice on cheap and effective ways of dealing with this is likely to give long-term benefits. Once the pharmacist has identified from questioning that the constipation is due to dietary causes, advice can be given about ways in which to increase fibre intake. However, it is nearly always the case that customers seeking a laxative from the pharmacist are likely to need relief from their uncomfortable symptoms quickly. There is no reason why the pharmacist should not recommend a laxative for short-term use to relieve the immediate problem. High-fibre foods are better introduced gradually into the diet, and increasing dietary fibre will take up to a week to improve gut motility and stool consistency.

Haemorrhoids (piles) are often caused by the straining which accompanies constipation, and the guidelines given above can be used to offer advice about reducing discomfort from haemorrhoidal symptoms associated with constipation and preventing their recurrence.

While it is outside the scope of this book to discuss the differentiation of symptom causation, it is important to emphasize that prolonged change in bowel habit in anyone aged over 50, particularly if accompanied by rectal bleeding, requires immediate medical referral. Bowel cancer is rare in those aged under 50 and commonly presents as a sustained change in bowel habit (particularly constipation).

Leaflets or other written information about the fibre content of specific foods can be most helpful. Encouraging customers to read food labels while shopping can also be helpful in identifying good sources of fibre. Local health promotion agencies have a range of leaflets on nutrition, which can be stocked by the pharmacist. One further point. Practising pharmacists are well aware of the misuse of laxatives by, mostly, young women with eating disorders. Newly qualified pharmacists need to be aware of the issue and the potential for encouragement to seek help.

8.5   Case studies

The opportunities for advice on healthy eating are interwoven everywhere into pharmacy practice. From the customer who complains of heartburn after meals to those complaining of constipation and haemorrhoids, there are opportunities everywhere for the pharmacist to offer good advice. To do so, pharmacists need to be informed on the key risk areas and also to recognize the important part that diet plays in the whole lifestyle.

Women form the majority of pharmacy customers, and it is largely they who determine what food will be bought for the family. But they must always strike a balance between good advice which may be given by the pharmacist and what their families will actually eat, ranging from pernickety children to husbands who are set in their dietary ways. Thus, the pharmacist will need to listen with care to what the customer says about the family's likes before deciding on key areas where change could be affected. Nor should the pharmacist forget the very real possibility of malnourishment as symptoms are being discussed particularly with elderly customers and/or those who have been bereaved, suffer from depression, or who have illnesses such as arthritis where food preparation can be a challenging task. A gentle reminder of the importance of regular meals and of possible help available, could be of great value.

1. *'My husband's just come out of the hospital. We've had such a fright—he had a heart attack. He's on tablets for his high blood pressure now but he's been told to cut down on fats and to lose some weight. He's 12 stones and should be 11 stones. Have you got any good diet sheets?'*
2. *'My husband's had his cholesterol done at the doctor's—it was over 7. How can he get it down? And should I change my diet as well?'*

Here the key issue is to check the advice given by the hospital and/or the GP. It is likely that they have been told to reduce saturated fat, and in the first case also to reduce salt. Care should be taken in supporting advice that customers are put onto a weight reduction diet only where needed. Where weight loss is not necessary, the amount of saturated fat should be reduced without calorie reduction by reducing the amount of dairy food and red meat, and poultry, fish, and carbohydrates (pulses, potatoes, and wholemeal bread) should be used as their replacement. Verbal advice should be supported by written material in the form of easily understood leaflets.

3. *'Well, here I am again. It's another April and I'm 2 stones overweight. I tried that micro diet last year and it really worked, so I suppose I'll try it again. What do you think?'*

Advice needs to be given with sensitivity here as to what is an achievable goal, bearing in mind the amount of pleasure that may be derived from a plate of chips or a cream cake. Where the pharmacy has facilities for weighing and measuring height, the body mass index (BMI) can be calculated and advice given accordingly. A person with a BMI of over 25 is generally considered as being 'overweight', and of over 30 as 'obese'. Weight reduction is best achieved by reduction in fat intake, particularly of saturated fat, and by reducing the amount of sugar that is eaten. The pharmacist should explain that starchy foods such as potatoes and pulses are filling and nutritious. Finally, but very importantly, taking more exercise will help in the weight loss programme. The pharmacist can keep a stock of weight recording sheets and can invite the customer to return to the pharmacy to monitor progress. Referral to the dietitian could be considered if the appropriate weight loss is not achieved.

4. *'But I can't afford it—these healthy foods are too expensive. And anyway I haven't got time.'*

Some of the recommended advice on better eating habits may mean higher expenditure on food. Several studies have shown that the diet of people living on unemployment benefit is likely to consist of a high percentage of processed food, tinned food, white bread, and high-sugar foods. The reasons are very simple: they are the cheapest to buy, the energy required to heat and serve them is very low, and they can be purchased locally—very important considerations for people who cannot afford bus fares to a supermarket. Nonetheless, there is much advice that can be offered to show, for example, that high-fibre foods need not be expensive, including potatoes, wholemeal bread (although this is always more expensive than white), and baked beans. Fat can also be reduced in cost-efficient ways such as the use of polyunsaturated spreads and semi-skimmed milk. Care should be taken that high-cost suggestions are not made to those on reduced incomes, such as baking potatoes in their jackets when no other foods are to be cooked in the oven, since high energy use and cost will result. However, while the microwave oven continues to make its appearance in large numbers of households with a range of incomes, a cheap and rapid way to cook potatoes in their jackets may be available. For working mothers who want to prepare meals quickly, tinned pulses are a good source of fibre and an alternative to the lengthy soaking and cooking process of raw pulses. These few examples show the way in which advice can be fitted to the individual customer.

5. *'What have you got for heartburn? I get it terribly after meals and when I go to bed.'*

Heartburn and gastro-oesophageal reflux are symptoms where health education advice is more important than treatment with over-the-counter medicines. Being overweight is a major cause of heartburn, and advice on weight reduction can be given where appropriate. General healthy eating advice is relevant—eating meals with a lower fat content will help to reduce the symptoms of heartburn by decreasing the length of time for which food remains in the stomach. Reducing alcohol intake can be helpful, since alcohol makes the sphincter between the stomach and oesophagus less effective. Smoking has a similar effect, and cutting down or stopping will lead to an improvement in the problem. While this, like alcohol consumption, can be a sensitive area to introduce into the conversation, the pharmacist can simply offer information in a non-judgemental way about the contribution which smoking and alcohol make to heartburn. Eating small meals often rather than the standard three meals each day means that the stomach is less full, and therefore its contents are less likely to leak back into the oesophagus. Finally, avoiding eating full meals within an hour or two of bedtime should help, and the pharmacist can supply antacid to help until the lifestyle measures begin to take effect.

References

Committee on Medical Aspects of Food Safety (1984) *Diet and Cardiovascular Disease.* HMSO, London.

Committee on Medical Aspects of Food Safety (1989) *Dietary Sugars and Human Disease.* HMSO, London.

Committee on Medical Aspects of Food Safety (1994) *Diet and Cardiovascular Disease.*

Committee on Medical Aspects of Food Safety (1998) *Nutritional Aspects of the Development of Cancer.*

Mason P. N. (1999) *Nutrition and Dietary Advice in the Pharmacy*, (2nd edn). Blackwell Science, Oxford.

Mason P. N. (1995) *Handbook of Dietary Supplements.* Blackwell Science, Oxford.

9 Physical activity

There is now compelling evidence that a sedentary lifestyle is detrimental to health. Indeed, the latest research shows that there are substantial benefits to be gained from a progression from no physical activity to even relatively low levels of physical activity. The health benefits of physical activity can be considered in terms of longevity, mortality and morbidity, psychological well-being, and social aspects (such as the ability to keep mobile and independent in old age). It is therefore important that pharmacists promote physical activity as part of their overall health promotion activities.

9.1 Definition of physical activity

Physical activity is a global term referring to any bodily movement produced by skeletal muscles that results in energy expenditure. It includes activities undertaken as part of daily life and work as well as activities such as exercise and sports. Exercise is planned, structured, involves repetitive bodily movements, and is usually undertaken during leisure time for the purpose of maintaining physical fitness. Physical fitness is a set of attributes that people have or can acquire that relates to their ability to perform physical activity. There are several components to physical activity, including aerobic fitness which relates to the ability of the heart and lungs to supply fuel during sustained physical activity and to eliminate waste products. Strength relates to the amount of external force that a muscle can exert and flexibility relates to the range of motion at a joint.

Intensity of physical activity must also be defined. Light activities require little exertion, not causing a noticeable change in breathing. Moderate activities require sustained, rhythmic, muscular movements at least the equivalent of brisk walking and leave someone feeling warm and slightly out of breath. Vigorous activity requires sustained, rhythmic, large muscle movements at a minimum of 60–70 per cent of heart rate and leaves someone sweating and out of breath.

Improvements in fitness and health depend not only on the intensity of physical activity but also on the duration and frequency of that activity. Current thinking on what constitutes a healthy level of activity is changing, and there is recognition that vigorous fitness training activity, while healthy in most cases, is not necessary for everyone. Indeed, there is increasing evidence that 10 minute exercise sessions are equally effective. The main dimension of physical activity that confers benefit is the volume of activity, irrespective of the duration of activity bouts, the number of activity bouts per week, and the possible intensity of the activity. The most dramatic reduction in risk is between the most sedentary individuals and those in the next lowest activity category. This is important when considering the health promotion messages that pharmacists might give. More moderate activity carries the majority of health benefits while being more sustainable.

The Department of Health published health-related activity guidelines for adults in 1996. The guidelines emphasize 30 min of moderate intensity (equivalent to brisk walking) activity on at least 5 days a week. This is a shift from the previous guidelines which emphasized more vigorous activity.

9.1.2 Prevalence of physical activity

Research shows that more people believe they are undertaking sufficient activity than is actually the case (see Table 9.1). In 1990–1, roughly only one-third of men and about one-quarter of women were undertaking regular moderate physical activity, although about half believed they were doing so.

Older people are more likely to lead a sedentary lifestyle than younger people. Most physical activity takes place in and around the home. A sedentary lifestyle is more likely to be linked to living in rented council accommodation than for those who own their own home. There is evidence that indicates an increase in population physical activity over the 10 years to 1995, although there is a

Table 9.1   Physical activity levels (actual and believed) of men and women aged between 16 and 74, 1990–1

	Men	Women
'Sedentary'	29%	28%
Are doing regular moderate activity	36%	24%
Believe they are doing sufficient moderate activity	56%	52%

marked decrease in the proportion of girls between the ages of 11 and 15 who take daily exercise.

9.2   The benefits of physical activity

Research has now shown convincingly that physical activity provides a range of health benefits, and these are summarized in Box 9.1.

9.2.1   Potential health gain from increased physical activity

If everyone adopted the recommended levels of physical activity, the overall gain in health would be:

- nearly one-third of all CHD incidence avoided
- one-quarter of stroke avoided
- nearly one-quarter of non-insulin-dependent diabetes in over 45 year olds avoided
- just over half the hip fractures in over 45 year olds avoided

(Source: *Health Update 5—Physical Activity*. Health Education Authority, 1995)

Coronary heart disease

Several population studies have shown lower mortality and increased longevity with high levels of physical activity or aerobic fitness. Many prospective studies have shown that regular physical

---

Box 9.1. Health benefits of physical activity

- lower mortality from all causes
- reduced risk of developing coronary heart disease
- reduced mortality after a heart attack
- reduced risk of heart attack in obese patients
- possible reduced risk of stroke
- lowering of high blood pressure
- greater weight loss than by dieting alone, and a better conservation of fat-free body tissue during dieting
- lower mortality from cancer of the colon
- lower incidence of non-insulin-dependent diabetes
- better management of insulin-dependent diabetes
- higher bone mass density and fewer osteoporotic fractures
- improved muscle strength and flexibility in elderly people
- reduction in mild anxiety and depression
- improved memory in elderly people
- improved self-esteem and confidence in performing daily tasks for elderly people

(Source: *Health Update 5—Physical Activity*. Health Education Authority, 1995)

---

activity is associated with a reduced risk of coronary heart disease (CHD). Indeed, physical activity seems to offer similar protection as not smoking or as not having high blood pressure. Most studies clearly indicate that the risk of CHD decreases with increasing physical activity. While the benefits of vigorous exercise are well recognized, there is a developing consensus that regular moderate activity will also confer health benefits. In addition, there is strong evidence that it is current physical activity that confers benefit for cardiovascular health, not previous activity in adult life.

It is likely that part of the mechanism by which physical activity protects against CHD is by modifying other CHD risk factors such as body weight, decreasing blood clotting, lowering blood pressure, producing a more favourable lipoprotein profile, and increasing insulin sensitivity. If obese people take regular exercise, they reduce their risk of heart disease to the same as that of exercisers of normal weight. Sedentary people who are obese have five times the risk of CHD. Physical activity programmes can also reduce the risk of mortality after heart attack by around 20 per cent.

Stroke

There is no clear cut evidence of a causal relationship between higher levels of physical activity and reduced risk of stroke. However, there is a strong association between inactivity and stroke. Physical activity may protect against stroke by modifying high blood pressure, a risk factor for stroke.

Cancer

Increased physical activity may prevent cancer development at several sites in the body. Much of the research has focused on cancer of the colon. A significant, inverse association between physical activity level and risk of colon cancer has been reported. The most inactive people have been found to have between 1.2 and 3.6 times the colon cancer risk of the most physically active.

Moderate exercise enhances the immune system and this may be linked to a reduced risk of cancer. Exercise fitness may also reduce reactivity to stress (psychosocial) and detoxify the effects of biochemical changes associated with the stress response. This may also be linked to a reduced cancer risk, but the evidence is not yet definitive.

Osteoporosis

In osteoporosis, low bone density and deterioration of bone mass tissue make the bones fragile and at greater risk of fracture. Osteoporosis results in about 6000 hip fractures a year in the UK. During the 10 years post-menopause, a gradual loss of bone mineral density occurs in both sexes, but is greater in women.

There is clear evidence that weight-bearing exercise helps to maintain bone mass and, in its absence (for example during bed rest or as a result of disability), there is a rapid decrease in bone density.

Active men and women have a higher bone density mass and less osteoporotic fractures than their inactive peers. However, it is not yet clear whether this is due to a direct effect on bone density or to the beneficial effects of exercise on muscle strength, balance, and coordination, helping to prevent the falls occurring in the first place. Regular physical activity, which is weight bearing (including walking), therefore has a significant part to play in reducing osteoporotic fractures (see also Chapter 12, Womens health).

Diabetes

There is evidence that physical activity helps to defer or prevent the development of non-insulin-dependent diabetes mellitus. For people who have developed insulin-dependent diabetes mellitus, increased physical activity appears to be protective against cardiovascular disease.

Weight control and obesity

Combined with dieting, regular physical activity is one of the most effective means of managing mild to moderate obesity. In overweight men and women, aerobic exercise causes a modest loss of weight even without dieting. When combined with dieting, exercise has been shown to achieve weight loss while conserving more fat-free body tissue than with dieting alone.

Mental health

Physical activity also has positive effects on mood, cognitive functioning, and quality of life. It therefore has an important role to play in anxiety and depression.

9.2.2 Maintaining health and mobility in later life

One of the main customer groups seen in pharmacies are the over-60s, and pharmacists are well placed to promote the benefits of exercise to this group. Physical activity has been shown to have many benefits in later life, including improvements in balance, coordination, mobility, strength, and endurance, as well as in the control of chronic diseases such as angina pectoris, heart failure, asthma, and chronic bronchitis, and in enhancing mental health.

Women aged 75–93, who were exercising three times a week for 12 weeks, increased their strength by 24–30 per cent. In relation to aerobic fitness, people who continue to exercise show less than expected deterioration with ageing. Even a modest programme of walking has been shown to improve aerobic fitness substantially for previously sedentary elderly people. In addition, recreational exercise offers opportunity for socializing, thus reducing the effects of isolation often experienced by the elderly.

9.2.3   Safety of physical activity

It is widely agreed that for stroke and CHD prevention, the benefits of physical activity far outweigh the risks as long as the intensity of activity is appropriate for the individual concerned. It should be aerobic and progressive to longer duration of activity (gradually over a number of weeks for those new or returning to physical activity). Recommendations for physical activity must be applicable to the individual, who should chose a form of exercise that suits them, so that a long-term behaviour change is more likely to result.

9.2.4   Measures to promote physical activity in the primary care setting

Many GPs have been involved in prescription for exercise, exercise referral, and walking for health programmes. Many of these have been linked to local sports and leisure centres. Numerous programmes and pilot schemes exist, but few have been evaluated rigorously. In 1998, the Health Education Authority (HEA) published a review of the published evidence and conducted three case studies of existing schemes. Published studies demonstrated a small improvement in physical activity patterns and other activity-related measures. Data from the case studies indicated considerable impact in a range of parameters and on a range of people.

In terms of promoting physical activity, people should be encouraged to take up walking and it should be made clear that in order to be active, people do not have to belong to a group, although support of this sort can help. For some people, the supervision and security of having an expert on hand can be an important motivating factor. Healthy Living Centres are likely to have an important role to play in future schemes to encourage physical activity. The HEA review showed that none of the schemes studied were based on existing models of behaviour change (see Chapter 4, How can behaviour be changed?). Expectations of such programmes must be realistic and, as in smoking cessation and weight loss programmes, changes in large numbers of participants are unlikely to occur.

9.2.5 Measures to promote physical activity in community pharmacy

Avon health authority and health promotion service examined the feasibility of promoting physical activity through community pharmacies. Fifteen pharmacies completed the project, in which they were trained and provided with specially developed shelf advertising resources. Further support was provided throughout the project, and the pharmacists were interviewed before and 4 months after the training. Seven customers had asked for advice following the training, compared with one before. The extent to which pharmacists gave unsolicited advice is more difficult to ascertain. Pharmacists reported that they were actively introducing the idea of more physical activity more often than they had before the training. Five of the pharmacists, prompted by GP prescriptions for certain medicines, had developed a targeted approach. They reported that they had concentrated on prescriptions for conditions where regular physical activity could be beneficial in its management or improvement, for example high cholesterol, diabetes, arthritis, and mobility problems.

It is important that pharmacists are aware of the factors that might encourage people to be more physically active. Research shows that people are motivated to take part in physical activity to feel in good shape, to improve and maintain health, to feel a sense of achievement, and to get out of doors. Other reasons include to have fun, to relax, and to control and lose weight. Over 40 per cent of men and women cite lack of time as the main barrier to them taking exercise. Twenty four per cent of men and 37 per cent of women say that not being 'sporty types' is a barrier. Qualitative research among South Asian and black communities has shown similar barriers to taking physical activity to those expressed by the population as a whole. However, barriers related to the use of facilities and outdoor recreation were prominent and more specific, and included dress codes and lack of separate male and female provision. Other perceptions included the fact that South Asians were not perceived to be physically strong enough to do competitive sport and that South Asian women were perceived to be housebound. Interestingly, the black community felt that because they were perceived to be fit they were sometimes paid less attention.

Motivational interviewing may be used to help people change their behaviour (see Chapter 4 for a fuller discussion on this aspect). People will be at various stages in their cycle of change, and different approaches should be taken during the interview dependent on the stage or readiness to change.

Pre-contemplation—'I am active enough to maintain good health'. The pharmacist can establish how active they actually are, ask if they could increase their activity, give information regarding the beneficial affects of exercise that is targeted to that patient's or customer's needs, illness, and so on.

Contemplation—The person accepts that they could be more active and recognizes the health benefits but needs to put this belief into reality. The pharmacist can explore reasons for change, reinforce positive feelings, and examine barriers, for example:

No time for exercise—advise to fit into normal routine, suggest walk or cycle to work, walk to the shops.

'Exercise makes me tired'—the pharmacist's response could be 'makes you less tired, try it and see'

Dislikes sport—could garden or walk

Dislikes communal activity—could walk or jog or use exercise machines

Dislikes exercising alone—could try dancing or a keep fit class.

Preparation—The person must make the decision to change. Pharmacists can give options for increased activity and help them to plan it.

Action—Remind the person that they should start gently and build up gradually, encourage them

Maintenance—Follow them up, ask how they are doing, encourage achievement, and recognize improvements, for example less tired, weight loss. Help them to set new goals

Relapse—Everyone relapses at some time and there are many reasons for this, for example changes in commitments, illness, holidays, weather. Encourage them to re-think their priorities and move back to action again

Pharmacists need to be aware of local services and facilities so that they can refer people for appropriate activities. They could set priorities to target certain customers and patients who are at a higher risk, for example those with a BMI more than 25, certain sex and age groups, and to provide population messages via leaflets, posters, and window displays for those at low or moderate risk and for passing trade.

9.3 Risks of increased physical activity

All the benefits of regular physical activity must be balanced against the risks. The main concerns are possible risks of heart attacks, accidents and injuries, and wear and tear of joints. Most problems arise when activity is extreme, when inadequate preparation is made, or when unfit people engage in heavy exertion and ignore the warning signs. Exercise-induced cardiac death is rare in the general population without underlying disease. Heavy physical exertion in unfit people is followed by a period of increased vulnerability to heart attack lasting about 24 hours. Fit people also show a slightly increased risk after very heavy, unaccustomed exercise. Musculo-skeletal injuries and accidents are also possible risks of physical activity.

9.3.1 Accidents and injuries

For walking and gardening, two of the most common activities, there is a low risk of musculoskeletal injuries. Research in 1998 showed that in the 22 million 16- to 45-year-olds, 19.2 million new injuries occur during sports and exercise each year, 5.1 million seek treatment, and a further 4.7 million have a resulting restriction in normal activities for at least one day. The highest death rates are found in air sports, water sports, climbing, and motor racing, followed at a lower level by horse riding and rugby. In 1993, there were 24 068 cycle casualties in Great Britain, of which 186 were fatal. The effectiveness of cycle helmets in reducing both death and severity of injuries has been demonstrated. Cycle helmets are now a legal requirement for cyclists in a number of countries including the USA.

Adverse effects of intense training have been reported for competitive athletes and performers. Increased training in children may delay the onset of puberty, and amenorrhoea has been reported in women athletes, the resulting low levels of oestrogen leading to more rapid loss of bone density. Indeed, if amenorrhoea continues for more than 2 years, this bone density loss may be irreversible and will increase the risk of osteoporosis in later life.

9.4   Case studies

1. A woman in her thirties asks your advice regarding weight control.

You discuss diet but also ask her how active she is. She tells you that she has a desk job and is usually too tired to do anything except sit in front of the TV in the evenings. She used to swim but it is too much effort. The pharmacist can offer advice about gradually increasing activity, walking to work if possible, walking at lunch time, and starting swimming again. She could be encouraged to go swimming on the way home from work, so that she is not tempted to sit in front of the TV instead. The woman can be encouraged by reassuring her that regular exercise combined with dieting will bring about a reduction in her weight.

2. A man presents a prescription for bendrofluazide 2.5 mg, he tells the pharmacist he has just been diagnosed with 'blood pressure'.

This is an ideal opportunity for the pharmacist to discuss physical activity with the man. He may have been already told by his GP to increase his activity, and the pharmacist can ask what, if anything, the doctor said about physical activity then reinforce this advice as well as encouraging him to be more active. Explain that 'even' just walking or gardening are effective forms of physical activity. The pharmacist can tell him that regular physical activity can help to reduce his blood pressure.

3. *A woman asks you if it is safe for her mother of 82 to take part in aerobic classes for the over-75s at her local leisure centre.*

These activities are usually tailored to the specific client so will probably be at a suitable level for a woman of 82. The woman should be encouraged to check the qualifications and training of the instructor to work with frail older people. Muscle strength and mobility are very important for older people in maintaining mobility for performing daily activities and avoiding further disability with ageing. Physical activity will help her to have better balance and coordination and she will be less likely to have falls.

References

Better Living. Better Life (1993) Knowledge House, Henley on Thames.
Health Education Authority (1995) *Health Update 5—Physical Activity.* Health Education Authority, London.
Health Education Authority (1998) *Promoting Physical Activity through Primary Healthcare: A Review.* Health Education Authority, London.
Riddoch. C., Puig-Ribera, A. and Cooper, A. (1998) *Effectiveness of Physical Activity Programmes in Primary Care: A Review.* Health Education Authority, London.

10 Oral health

Giving oral health advice is an important role for pharmacists as they sell a wide range of dental health-related products. A large number of the population do not visit the dentist unless they are in pain, and many of these consult a pharmacist first. However, dentists often criticize pharmacists for giving mixed messages about oral health because they stock confectionery, fizzy drinks, sugar-containing baby foods and drinks, and do not always recommend sugar-free medicines.

The results of a 1996 postal survey of community pharmacists in a South London health authority showed that the majority were knowledgeable about dental caries and felt they had a role in oral health promotion; 92 per cent said that they always recommended sugar-free medicines. The pharmacists estimated that advice was sought about dental health at least 1–5 times a week.

10.1 The problems

Dental caries (tooth decay) in children and periodontal (gum) disease in adults are the most common dental problems. Of the UK's 5-year-olds, 45 per cent have teeth that are decayed or have been extracted or filled because of decay. Tooth decay is higher in children from lower social classes, the North of England and Scotland, and in Bangladeshi and Pakistani ethnic groups. Dental erosion by acidic drinks, such as fizzy drinks and fruit juice, and other sources of acid now affects 30 per cent of 13-year-olds. Oral cancer is a problem in adults and is linked to smoking, alcohol consumption and, in some ethnic groups, betel nut chewing. Early detection is important.

10.1.1 The decay process

Decay is caused by the interaction of sugar and dental plaque. A layer of plaque, largely made up of bacteria, forms continuously on the tooth surface. Each time sugar enters the mouth, the plaque bacteria metabolize it and produce acid as a by-product. While the plaque is acidic, it dissolves minerals (calcium and phosphate) from the surface of the teeth—demineralization. The plaque layer stays acidic until saliva neutralizes the acid. This takes about half an hour and remineralization takes place. If demineralization is not balanced out by remineralization, a cavity will form.

10.1.2 Erosion

Erosion is decay caused by non-bacterial attack on the teeth. The acids that cause erosion come mainly from acid drinks, such as fizzy colas and fruit drinks and including diet drinks, from sucking citrus fruits, from frequent vomiting, for example in bulimia or anorexia, or from gastric reflux. The whole tooth surface is attacked, particularly the inside surface of the upper incisor teeth.

10.1.3 Periodontal disease

The first sign of periodontal disease is inflammation of the gums, indicated by redness, swelling, and bleeding. This is called gingivitis and is caused by plaque that is not removed by effective brushing. Plaque remaining at the tooth gum margin is the largest problem, so people should be encouraged to brush their gums as well as their teeth. Just over a quarter of 5-year-olds and almost two-thirds of 10-year-olds as well as a large proportion of the adult population have gingivitis. Gingivitis is reversible with good oral hygiene; peridontitis, however, which is the next stage in gum disease, produces permanent damage, It involves inflammation and destruction of the tooth's attachment to the jawbone. This is followed by the loss of supporting bone itself. Peridontitis occurs mainly in adults.

10.1.4 Oral cancer

About 2500 new case of malignant tumours of oral epithelium are reported in England and Wales every year, with 300 malignancies of the salivary gland. Many cases are smoking or alcohol related, a combination of both multiplying the risk. Chewing betel nut quid-containing tobacco is also a risk factor. This is most common among older Bangladeshi men and women. Oral cancers often present as symptomlesss ulcers, commonly around the tongue. If someone has had an ulcer for more than 2–3 weeks, a screening visit with a general dental practitioner is essential. Another symptom is ulceration with a pre-existing white or thickened area of mucous. Tumours of the salivary gland or bone usually take the form of swellings.

10.2   Dental health promotion

The HEA recommended in 1996 that dental health education advice should be based on four statements involving diet, toothbrushing, fluoridation, and visits to the dentist.

10.2.1   Diet

Dietary sugars can be divided into two groups:

Intrinsic sugars—form an integral part of whole fruit and vegetables; as they are enclosed in the cellular structures of the food, they do not cause tooth decay.

Extrinsic sugars—are those not found in the cellular structure of food. Milk sugars (mainly lactose) are extrinsic sugars but are much less likely to cause decay than other extrinsic sugars. The sugars that cause decay are table sugar, sugars added to food during manufacture, fruit juices with added sugar, and honey. The Department of Health recommends that the average intake of non-milk sugars should be no more than 10 per cent of total energy intake. The current intake of pre-school children is about twice that.

The number of times that sugar enters the mouth is the most important factor in determining rate of decay. Sweets should be consumed as part of a meal rather than as a snack, this is because salivary flow is higher at this time and recovery from an acid attack is quicker. Snacks and drinks should be sugar free, and the frequent consumption of acidic drinks should be avoided.

10.2.2   Toothbrushing

People should be advised to clean their teeth and gums thoroughly twice each day with a fluoride-containing toothpaste. Plaque removal is essential for prevention of periodontal disease Toothbrushing is the most effective method of plaque removal. Thorough brushing twice a day is more effective than frequent cursory brushing; gentle scrub techniques should be advised. Toothbrushing by itself will not reduce dental decay, but a major benefit will be gained by use of a fluoride toothpaste. Vigorous toothbrushing after exposure to an acid may worsen erosion. Dentists recommend toothbrushing about an hour after exposure to acid.

10.2.3 Fluoridation

Fluoride is absorbed by plaque and the surface enamel of the tooth, reducing acid production from sugars and promoting remineralization. This is a topical effect. Frequent small doses of fluoride are more effective than occasional high doses. Fluoride is also absorbed systemically into the tooth as it forms. Systemic fluoride is less significant in preventing decay than topical fluoride. Excessive intake of fluoride can result in faint white marks on the surface of the teeth, called mottling. The major cause of fluoride-induced mottling is excessive blood fluoride when the crowns of the front teeth are forming, at between 1 and 5 years of age. The risk of mottling is negligible if the child does not swallow excessive quantities of fluoride. A tiny smear of toothpaste is sufficient for an infant, and a pea size blob for children. Mottling can be caused by giving children fluoride drops when there is already fluoride in the water supply. Fluoride-containing toothpaste is the main reason for the decline in caries in the last 20 years.

The use of fluoride supplements is not a normal public health measure, although their use may be of value in areas where the dental health of pre-school children is poor. Supplements can be taken daily in areas where the fluoride levels in drinking water are low, that is below 0.7 p.p.m. Pharmacists can check with their local general dental practitioners or their local water board to ascertain the local fluoride levels. Appropriate use depends on a professional assessment of the likely benefit, and recommended dosages are reviewed periodically by expert groups. Fluoride supplements are licensed medicinal products and the manufacturer's recommended dosage appears on product labels and in the *British National Formulary*.

If supplements are to be taken, tablets which can be sucked or chewed are more effective because of the additional topical effect. Care should be taken that the dose is not inflated by additional liberal use of fluoride toothpaste. If a dose or supplement is missed one day it should not be made up by doubling the dose the next day. The benefit of maternal fluoride to children is small, so there is little point in pregnant women taking fluoride supplements, as has been advocated by some.

10.2.4 Dental attendance

Everyone, irrespective of age and dental condition, should have an oral examination once a year. NHS check-ups and advice are free to all children under the age of 18, those under 19 in full-time education, those receiving income support or family credit, and pregnant women or those who have a child under 1 year. Children and those at risk from oral disease may need to be seen more frequently. The community dental service is responsible for carrying out dental screening in schools and in homes for the elderly, and offering care to special needs adults and children. Pharmacists could work together with local general dental practitioners on local dental health campaigns. Team work ensures that the same messages are being given out by all professionals, and the more professionals who are giving a particular message the more reinforcement of that message takes place. Most health authorities have a public dental health adviser or consultant, they will usually be glad to offer support.

10.2.5 Health promotion themes

There are a number of health promotion themes that could be followed.

Advice on diet

Diet and dental health could be the focus for an event in pharmacies, displays could be put up on a board in the pharmacy or in pharmacy windows. Messages could include the importance of avoiding sugary and acidic drinks, not dipping babies dummies in sugar, the fact that 'hidden sugar' is contained in many foods, and avoiding sugar-containing snacks but rather eating sweets as part of meals. Parents can be informed that babies can be conditioned not to acquire a preference for sweetened foods by giving completely unsweetened baby drinks. Herbal baby drinks, especially those with a fruit component, have an acidogenic potential, they may also have an erosive potential, and all have cariogenic potential.

Advice on medicines

Pharmacists should encourage local GPs not to prescribe sugar-containing medicines especially for the medically compromised and chronically sick children. Sugar-free alternatives exist for most prescription and over-the-counter medicines; if a sugar-containing medicine is unavoidable, it should be given at a mealtime and the teeth should be brushed immediately afterwards. Pharmacists should consider only stocking sugar-free formulations of over-the-counter products. Many children unnecessarily go on taking liquid formulations as they get older, and they can take tablets or capsules at an earlier age than they usually do.

Toothbrushing

Brushing the teeth is often performed in a perfunctory fashion with benefit probably perceived as a result of freshening the mouth from the flavouring in the toothpaste, rather than any real cleaning of the teeth. However, if toothbrushing is carried out twice a day, using the correct technique, and with a suitable toothbrush and tooth-paste, it is the cornerstone of preventive dental care. Toothbrushes, toothpaste, and so on could be merchandized near to the medicines counter with notices attached saying the pharmacist will advise about their use. Leaflets and posters about their correct use can also be displayed.

Fluoride

All pharmacies stock toothpaste and can place leaflets about use of fluoride-containing toothpastes where toothpaste is displayed.

Fluoride is more effective via its topical effect on the enamel and plaque rather than systemically using fluoride drops or tablets.

Many dentists now recommend topical use via toothpaste, rather than systemic treatment, for children. This is partly because children tend to swallow toothpaste and so get an additional systemic effect from their daily brushing routine.

Dental attendance

Pharmacists are ideally placed to encourage those who never visit a dentist to do so. In some parts of the country, NHS dentists are hard to find and local lists could be held in the pharmacy. Pharmacists could also hold details of emergency dental services in the area. An event could take place in the pharmacy to encourage people to visit the dentist. A local general dental practitioner or hygienist could come to the pharmacy and do check-ups in a different environment. A number of community pharmacists now rent out part of their premises to other health professionals, including dentists.

10.2.6   Guidelines for team working in dental health promotion

Guidelines for team working were produced by the Postgraduate Medical Department at the University of Dundee. The guidelines acknowledged the importance of other health professionals besides general dental practitioners in the prevention of dental caries. Pharmacists are encouraged to display leaflets on diet and tooth care, to contact their local GPs if they are consistently prescribing sugar-containing medicines, and to stock only sugar-free sweets.

A health authority pharmacy health promotion event on oral health

In a typical event, pharmacists will be asked to record enquires, advice, and sales of toothpaste, toothbrushes, toothache tinctures, ulcer treatments, and other oral health-related sales in a log for a 1-month period prior to the campaign. Pharmacists will be provided with uniform display materials for the event, and will continue to keep their log during the campaign and for a month afterwards.

Client surveys will be performed before and during the campaign to gauge the publics' acceptance of oral health promotion by community pharmacists, and those customers who seek advice will be followed up to see if they have acted on the advice. Toothbrush and toothpaste sales and dental consultations will be monitored across the health authority from supermarkets as well as pharmacies, before, during, and after the event.

10.3 Case studies

1. A mother asks you if you sell soft toothbrushes. She tells you that her 8-year-old daughter's gums are bleeding when she brushes her teeth.

Her daughter probably has gingivitis; it is nothing to do with the toothbrush. The pharmacist needs to discuss effective plaque removal with the mother and daughter, if she is there. Disclosing tablets can be a useful aid to plaque removal. The child should be taught to brush her gums as well as her teeth. The mother should be encouraged to take her daughter for a dental check-up. The pharmacist should warn her that bleeding may persist for up to 2 weeks as she recovers, but that if it persists she should consult her dentist or doctor as something more sinister like neutropenia or anaemia may be occurring.

2. A young mother who is handing over some milk tokens in exchange for formula baby milk asks the pharmacist why her 2-year-old daughter's teeth are already bad.

The pharmacist notices that the child has a dummy and also has chocolate stains around her mouth. This child is suffering from tooth decay; the mother should be encouraged to only give her sugar-containing foods with meals and to use other foods for snacks if snacks are necessary. The pharmacist should also check if the woman dips the child's dummy in honey or sugar and if she gives her sugary, acidic drinks. Regular toothbrushing with a fluoride-containing toothpaste and dental check-ups should be encouraged. The woman should be encouraged to make a dental appointment as soon as possible.

3. A 60-year-old man who regularly purchases smokers toothpaste asks the pharmacist for advice about a lump that has developed under his dentures; it has been there for about a month.

The man should be told to see his dentist straight away as the swelling could be a tumour. In order not to frighten the patient, the

pharmacist will need to carefully word a statement about why
seeing the dentist is important.

*4. A regular customer telephones and asks about emergency dental
treatment, she is in pain.*

The pharmacist ascertains that the woman is not registered with a
dentist. This may cause problems out of hours; pharmacists should
know about their health authority's provision of out of hours
dental services.

Further reading

Anderson, C. and Nathan, A. (1991) Promoting oral health. *Pharmaceutical Journal* 247, 734–736.

Davies, R. M., Holloway, P. J. and Ellwood, R. P. (1995). The role of
fluoride dentifrices in a national strategy for the oral health of children.
British Dental Journal 179, 84–87.

Department of Health (1994) *An Oral Health Strategy for England.* HMSO,
London.

Duggal, M. S., Toumba, K. J., Davies, R. M., Holloway, P. J. *et al.* (1996)
The role of fluoride dentifrices in a national strategy for the oral health
of children. *British Dental Journal* 180, 98–103.

Gregory, J. R., Collins, D. L., Davies, P. S. W. *et al.* (1995) *National Diet
and Nutrition Survey: Children one-and-a-half to four-and-a-half years.*
HMSO, London.

Health Education Authority (1996) *The Scientific Basis of Dental Health
Education,* (4th edn). Health Education Authority, London.

Health Education Authority (1998) *Oral Health Promotion: A Practical
Guide for Health Visitors and School Nurses.* Health Education
Authority, London.

11   Contraception and sexual health

One in three of all pregnancies in the UK is unplanned. Traditionally, the pharmacy has always been a major outlet for the sale and supply of contraceptives. Given the problems of privacy in the pharmacy, the number of people who ask directly for advice about contraception is small. However, the pharmacy is a good point from which to distribute information, in the form of leaflets, about contraceptives and about safer sex. The availability of such leaflets, together with the generally reduced extent to which Family Planning Clinics operate in some areas because of financial cuts in the NHS, mean that the community pharmacist is being asked for advice on a great number of occasions. Pharmacists, therefore, need to be well informed about contraceptive methods and about pregnancy and ovulation testing. In this chapter, we will consider the main methods of contraception and the type of questions that pharmacy customers may ask about them.

11.1   Contraceptive methods

There are 13 main forms of contraception.

- Oral contraceptive pills—combined pills, progestogen-only pills
- Barrier methods—male and female condoms, diaphragms, and caps
- Intra-uterine devices (previously known as 'the coil')
- Injectables
- Hormonal intra-uterine systems
- Hormonal implants
- 'Natural' birth control
- Female sterilization and male vasectomy

11.1.1   Oral contraceptive

These are of two main types: the combined oral contraceptive and the progestogen-only pill.

The combined oral contraceptive

The combined oral contraceptive is highly effective against pregnancy and works mainly by suppressing ovulation. Method failure rates are less than 1 pregnancy per 100 woman years. User failure rates depend on how well it is taken. Over the years, the relative doses of oestrogen and progestogen in the combined pill have been reduced. Most products require the pill to be taken for 3 weeks, with a 1-week break in which a withdrawal bleed occurs. There are three types of combined pills—monophasic (a fixed dose of oestrogen and progestogen), biphasic, and triphasic. The biphasic pill has one dosage change and the triphasic two such changes. The bi- and triphasic pills were developed to mimic cyclical hormonal changes. Bi- and triphasic pills may cause less inter-menstrual bleeding so might be tried if this has occurred with a monophasic pill, once all other factors have been checked. Everyday (ED) pills have 21 active and seven inactive pills.

There has been a great deal of negative publicity about adverse effects from the combined pill and, in particular, there has been concern about the dose of oestrogen within it. A pill with the lowest possible effective dose of oestrogen is now prescribed.

Taking the combined pill gives a protective effect against ovarian cancer, and against endometrial cancer and fibroids. Epidemiological studies have shown that bone loss, pelvic inflammatory disease, and ectopic pregnancy rates are lower in users of the combined pill.

Use of the combined pill has, however, been linked to an increased risk of heart disease and a possible increased risk of breast cancer and cervical cancer. Additionally, and in extremely rare cases, combined pill use has been linked to cancer of the liver, but the findings of studies have been conflicting. The risk–benefit ratio of taking the combined pill must be carefully considered by the woman and her prescriber. The risk of circulatory problems and, in particular, cerebrovascular events is greatly increased in women of all ages who smoke and those in older age groups. For women who are aged 35 or over and are smokers, the combined pill should be discontinued. In non-smokers, the combined pill can be continued until at least the age of 45. Pharmacists need to be aware that migraine-type headaches in women taking the combined pill can sometimes be a warning of cerebrovascular changes. Such women should be referred to their doctor. The findings of the long-term Royal College of General Practitioners study on oral contraception published in January 1999 shows negligible side-effects for women where they are selected appropriately.

Drugs such as rifampicin and phenytoin, which induce liver enzymes, may speed up metabolism of oestrogen and progestogen and make the pill ineffective. More controversial is the interaction between the pill and antibiotics. Here broad-spectrum antibiotics disturb the bacterial flora of the gut and prevent the reabsorption of oestrogen. The effect is on oestrogen and not progestogen, and ampicillin and tetracyclines are the drugs cited most commonly. Use of an additional contraceptive method should be advised. Low-dose tetracyclines in acne have not been reported to cause problems.

Prolonged or severe diarrhoea and vomiting may prevent full absorption of the contents of the combined pill and reduce its effectiveness. Diarrhoea can occur as a side-effect of a broad-spectrum antibiotic. If the woman has diarrhoea and vomiting either in association with an antibiotic or independently, additional contraception should be taken for as long as the diarrhoea lasts and for 7 days afterwards. If these 7 days overlap with the pill-free or inactive pill week, then the next pack should be started straight away without any break.

The combined pill should be stopped 1 month before planned major surgery (or where immobilization is an issue) to minimize the risk of post-operative thrombosis. The woman can start taking the pill again when she is fully mobile (usually at about 2 weeks after the operation) or at her next period.

The progestogen-only pill

The progestogen-only pill (POP, used to be called the 'mini-pill') must be taken regularly and within 3 hours of the same time each day, and thus requires a high degree of motivation. The pill is taken every day without a break and each pill gives some 27 hours protection. The POP works mainly by altering the production of cervical mucus, making it more difficult for sperm to reach the egg. Ovulation stops in 40 per cent of cycles in women taking the POP.

The effect of the POP on cervical mucus is at its minimum each time a dose is taken, but is still effective. Many women on this type of pill experience irregular periods and breakthrough bleeding, although their cycle often becomes more regular after a few months. Some women find that their periods become lighter, and others report that they have no periods at all.

The POP has a higher method failure rate than does the combined pill (1–2 per cent). If pill taking is delayed by longer than 3 hours, contraceptive protection may be lost. Broad-spectrum antibiotics do not interact with the POP but enzyme-inducing drugs do.

'Missed' pills

Women sometimes consult the pharmacist, explaining that they have 'missed' a pill and asking if they might be pregnant or whether they should use additional contraceptive methods and, if so, for how long. The risk of breakthrough ovulation is highest at the beginning or end of a pack of combined pills. The advice of the FPA is as follows.

For combined pills:

If you forget to take a pill, take it as soon as you remember, and the next one at your normal time. If you are 12 or more hours late with any pill (especially the first or last in the packet), the pill may not work. As soon as you remember, continue normal pill-taking. However, you will not be protected for the next 7 days and must either not have sex or use another method, such as the condom. If these 7 days run beyond the end of your packet, start the next packet at once, when you have finished the present one, i.e. do not have a time interval between packets. This will mean you may not have a period until the end of two packets but this does you no harm. Nor does it matter if you see some bleeding on pill-taking days. If you are using every day (ED) pills, miss out the seven inactive pills. If you are not sure which these are, ask your doctor.

For the progestogen-only pill:

If you forget to take a pill, take it as soon as you remember, and carry on with the next pill at the right time. If the pill is more than three hours overdue, you are not protected. Continue normal pill-taking but you must also use another method, such as the condom, for the next 7 days. If you have vomiting, or very severe diarrhoea, the pill may not work. Continue to take it, but you may not be protected from the first day of the vomiting or diarrhoea. Use another method, such as the condom, for any intercourse during the stomach upset and for the next 7 days.

Emergency contraception

Emergency contraception (sometimes called post-coital contraception) is a safe and effective way of preventing an accidental pregnancy after unprotected intercourse or a contraceptive accident. There are two types: hormonal methods or the insertion of a copper intra-uterine device (IUD). The most widely used hormonal preparation previously has been a combined oestrogen–progestogen regimen (the Yuzpe method). Each tablet contains 250 mcg of levonorgestrel and 50 mcg of ethinyloestradiol, available as the licensed product Schering PC4. Two tablets are taken as soon as possible after intercourse and not later than 72 hours after intercourse, the other two tablets after a further 12 hours. The treatment must be initiated within 3 days of having unprotected sex, but the earlier the better. The method is effective but the high dose of oestrogen which is consumed may cause nausea and even vomiting. Up to 50 per cent of women will experience nausea, and an anti-emetic is sometimes prescribed for this reason. Domperidone 10 mg has been used and is taken at the same time or just before each dose of emergency contraception. Up to 20 per cent of women will experience vomiting after taking emergency contraception. If vomiting occurs within 2 hours of the first dose, the woman should be referred back to the prescriber. Following post-coital contraception, the woman's period may begin on time or a little earlier or later than anticipated. The Yuzpe method has been shown to prevent at least three out of four pregnancies.

Another method using progestogen (levonorgestrel) alone (the Ho and Kwan method) has been shown in clinical trials to be more effective than the Yuzpe method. Nausea and vomiting were less likely to occur with the progestogen-only treatment (23 and 6 per cent, respectively). Both treatments were more effective the earlier they were given. A licensed levornorgestrel product for emergency contraception is expected to become available in the UK in 1999. It is likely that the levonorgestrel regimen will become widely used because of its increased efficacy and reduced side-effects. Furthermore, it can be used in women in whom the Yuzpe method might have been contra-indicated (migraine at presentation and previous history of migraine with aura; or past history of thrombo-embolism).

Anxieties have been expressed about the repeated use of the Yuzpe method for two reasons. The first is that repeat users may be seeking to use this as a method of contraception. Prescribers will make a decision about each individual case. However, the risk of pregnancy associated with emergency contraceptive use is higher than for established regular contraceptive use. The second concern is about safety and the likelihood that side-effects may occur. The hormonal dose in the Yuzpe treatment is equivalent to no more than seven pills of a low-dose combined pill, so concerns about adverse effects are unnecessary.

Pharmacists occasionally have been asked to supply post-coital contraception as an 'emergency supply'. Such a supply must be made under the provisions of the Medicines Act and the pharmacist will use their professional judgement in deciding whether this course of action will be taken. The Royal Pharmaceutical Society's Law Department reminds pharmacists of the requirements for such a supply: they are that the pharmacist must establish that the patient has been prescribed the treatment on a previous occasion. The pharmacist should also attempt to contact the prescriber in order to confirm the supply. If this is not possible, the pharmacist should strongly advise the patient to inform the prescriber of the supply. With the patient's agreement, the pharmacist may later inform the prescriber that the emergency supply was made.

It has been suggested that the legal category of the existing combined emergency hormonal contraception preparation (Yuzpe method) should be changed from Prescription Only to become a Pharmacy medicine. There has been much debate about this proposal in the pharmaceutical press, with strong feelings and arguments being demonstrated both for and against.

In an alternative form of emergency contraception, a copper IUD is fitted. The device should be fitted as soon as possible after unprotected intercourse, and within 5 days. Where the unprotected intercourse was more than 5 days previously, an IUD can be fitted up to 5 days after the calculated earliest day of ovulation. IUDs are highly effective and have the advantage of being used as an ongoing method of contraception.

11.1.2 Barrier methods

Condoms (Sheath)

The increasing incidence of sexually transmitted diseases including HIV and AIDS has led to greater use of condoms, and the 1980s and 1990s have seen a revival in popularity of this form of contraception. The use of condoms is a central feature of advice on safer sex. Only those condoms which have BSI (British Standards Institute) 'Kite Mark' approval (European mark BS EN 600) should be stocked, since these will have been tested and found to meet a particular standard. Customers who buy condoms will sometimes also wish to purchase a spermicidal gel or lubricant. All the spermicides on the market are compatible with condoms. Whilst water-based lubricants can be used with condoms, oil-based products are incompatible, so that petroleum jelly and baby or other oils should not be used with latex condoms but can be used with polyurethane types (male and female types). Polyurethane male and female condoms do not yet carry a BS EN 600 mark. Present figures for the contraceptive effectiveness of condoms show 85–98 per cent reliability. It is important to dispel the myth that condoms are not effective; condoms can only be as good as their user.

Caps and diaphragms

These prevent the passage of sperm into the womb. The cervical cap is held in place by suction and comes in three shapes and in a range of sizes. Prescribing of these is best done by a trained family planning professional, as is also the case with diaphragms. The diaphragm is also made of rubber but is kept in place by a pliable metal rim which is covered in rubber. There are three different types. If a woman complains of discomfort from a cap or diaphragm, refitting may be needed. Once a woman knows her size, she can buy caps and diaphragms from the pharmacist. Some pharmacists seem to be unaware of this and may unnecessarily refer women to their doctor or Family Planning Clinic. Caps and diaphragms also provide some protection against sexually trans-mitted diseases and appear to give some protection against cancer of the cervix.

A spermicide must be used with both the cap and diaphragm, and the device should be left in place for at least 6 hours after inter-course but removed within 30 hours. Contrary to popular opinion, the diaphragm can be inserted at any time before intercourse. If, however, intercourse occurs more than 3 hours after inserting the diaphragm, then a further application of spermicide should be used. Since these devices are made of rubber, only water-based spermi-cides should be used.

Advice about cleaning caps and diaphragms is given in the leaflets supplied with the devices. General rules are that unscented soap should be used in order to prevent irritant reactions and that the device should be left to dry. Caps and diaphragms should not be boiled, nor should they be cleaned with disinfectant, bleach, detergent, or any other chemical. Women should be aware that if their body weight changes by more than 3 kg (7 lbs), a differ-ent size of cap may be needed. A woman who has recently had a baby, miscarriage, or abortion will also probably require a different size.

Used carefully, caps and diaphragms can provide a high rate of contraceptive effectiveness (85–98 per cent) and a spermicide should always be used.

11.1.3   Intra-uterine devices (IUDs)

IUDs are fitted into the uterus and usually consist of a plastic moulding which is coated with thin copper wire. Advantages of the method are that it is effective immediately after insertion and provides long-term protection (5–10 years). The fpa's policy is that IUDs need not generally be changed more often than every 5 years, and the contraceptive efficacy of some devices has been shown to be far longer than 5 years. They do not need to be changed if inserted after the age of 40.

However, IUDs are not suitable for all women. IUDs are not recommended for women who are not in mutually faithful relationships. Infection associated with IUDs relates to lifestyle issues and not to the IUD. Contrary to myth, young women and women who have not had children can use IUDs when selected appropriately. Sometimes the IUD is expelled soon after insertion. It is recommended that, about 6 weeks after insertion, a check is done to ensure the IUD is in place, is sited correctly, and that there are no problems. Sometimes IUDs may cause heavier, longer, and more painful periods in some women. This is less of a problem with newer devices. Any pain at times other than menstruation, or signs of systemic infection such as feverishness, or vaginal discharge, would warrant immediate referral to the doctor.

11.1.4 Progestogen-releasing intra uterine systems (IUSs)

IUDs have been developed which contain progestogen and which release this gradually. The mechanism of action is similar to that of the other progestogen-only contraceptives. In addition to its effect on cervical mucus, it probably also has a modifying effect on ovulatory function. The physical presence of the device has only a minor contribution to its contraceptive effect. As with other progestogen-only methods, the progestogen-containing IUS can cause menstrual irregularities. After the first 3 months, the number of bleeding days and menstrual blood loss are reduced. In some countries, the device is licensed for the treatment of menorrhagia. Women using this method need to know that their periods may become less frequent or may stop altogether (amenorrhoea) but that this does not mean that they are pregnant. The normal menstrual pattern will be resumed after the device is removed. The IUS is highly effective and lasts for 5 years.

11.1.5 Injectables

Injectable contraceptives contain progestogens and are usually given as 'depot' formulations which will have a long-term action. Of the two products currently used in the UK, injections are needed at

8-weekly (Noristerat) or 12-weekly (Depo Provera) intervals. The injectables work in the same way as the progestogen-only pill but the high serum levels also inhibit ovulation. Advantages of this form of contraception are its effectiveness (less than 1 per cent failure) and that the method does not rely on memory, unlike pill-taking. However, side-effects are common. Some women find they have fewer periods and some become amenorrhoeic and have no periods at all. Others find that their periods become heavier, at least initially. Weight gain and depression have been reported as side-effects of this method of contraception.

Injectable methods are generally not recommended for women who wish to start a family in the near future, since their effect is cumulative and, even after stopping the injections, it may be a minimum of 9–10 months or longer before pregnancy is achieved (mainly Depo Provera related).

11.1.6 Implants

Progestogen implants provide a constant, continuous release of the hormone, giving an advantage over oral and injectable forms where greater plasma level fluctuations occur. The mode of action of implants is similar to that of injectables (see above). One of the advantages of an implant is that, unlike an injectable contraceptive, it can be removed if needed. Like other progestogen-only contraceptives, implants may cause menstrual irregularities.

Norplant, containing levornorgestrel in the form of six flexible silastic capsules, was launched early in the 1990s with the potential to provide contraceptive protection for up to 5 years. The implant was inserted under the skin of the upper arm through a small incision. Single-rod implants are being introduced such as Implanon. Releasing etonorgestrel, it is highly effective, with data showing no pregnancies to date. Implanon lasts for 3 years.

11.1.7 Natural methods (or fertility awareness methods)

Natural methods of contraception (formerly known as the 'rhythm' method) are based on signs and symptoms in the body which indicate ovulation and, therefore, the fertile time. Becoming familiar with how natural family planning works allows a couple to either plan a pregnancy or avoid conception. The methods involve careful recording of the signs and the keeping of records. The fertile period lasts for some 7 days—5 days before ovulation and at least 2 days afterwards, because sperm are viable for up to 7 days in the vagina. There are several different natural family planning indicators which allow a woman to observe the naturally occurring signs and symptoms of the fertile and infertile phases of the menstrual cycle.

If natural family planning is practised by a highly motivated couple who are well taught and committed to the method and will practise it carefully and conscientiously, then it is effective. Under these circumstances, of 100 women using the method for a year, only two will become pregnant (using multiple indicators). Should the method not be followed carefully, the effectiveness is reduced.

Many pharmacies stock fertility thermometers (mercury and digital) and temperature recording charts, together with their instructions. If the woman has not received explanation about how to use the natural method of contraception, then the details need to be outlined by the pharmacist and referral to a recognized centre teaching natural family planning is essential. A private area in the pharmacy is obviously necessary for such a consultation to take place.

11.1.8 Female sterilization and male vasectomy

Where a couple have completed their family or are sure that they do not want to have children, female sterilization or vasectomy for the male may be requested. For all practical purposes, these procedures should be regarded as irreversible. Occasionally, reversal operations are carried out but there are difficulties involved and the procedure may not be a success.

A vasectomy is carried out as a minor operation usually under local anaesthetic. After making small cuts in the scrotum, the vas deferens are cut and sealed. While sexual intercourse can be resumed as soon as the discomfort has ceased, it is important that other methods of contraception are used initially. There may still be active sperm present, and semen tests should always be carried out to check for this. Two clear semen tests must be produced before the vasectomy becomes a totally effective method of contraception. The failure rate is 1 in 2000.

Female sterilization is a more invasive and larger operation than is a vasectomy, and may involve a light general anaesthetic or a local anaesthetic. The fallopian tubes are either cut or blocked in order to prevent eggs travelling from the ovaries to the uterus. Following a female sterilization, additional contraceptive measures are always advised until the next menstrual period. The failure rate is 1 in 2000.

11.2   Pregnancy and ovulation testing

Home pregnancy testing kits are sold from pharmacies and, in addition, many pharmacies offer a pregnancy testing service. The accuracy of home testing kits is extremely high. In providing a pregnancy testing service, the pharmacist must comply with the Royal Pharmaceutical Society's guidelines (RPSGB Medicines and Ethics). As with any other diagnostic or screening test, the product and method used must be of a high level of accuracy, and the pharmacist or member of staff who carries out the test must be trained in its use and the interpretation of the results. The communication of the results of the test to the client must be done in an atmosphere of privacy and using great tact. Often the pharmacist has no way of knowing whether the woman might be desperate to have a child or whether becoming pregnant might be regarded as a disaster. Research in pharmacies has shown that around two-thirds of women who buy a home pregnancy testing kit want the result to be positive and that the commonest age group for women buying such kits is between 25 and 34 years, accounting for two-thirds of all pregnancy test kits purchased.

11.2.1   Test accuracy

The test detects the presence of human chorionic gonadotrophin (hCG). Such tiny amounts can be detected that some tests claim that a result can be obtained before the first missed period. However, the pharmacist must remember that almost two-thirds of pregnancies spontaneously miscarry within the first 20 days after implantation. In fact, what a woman might previously have thought to be a late period could indeed be an early pregnancy which has miscarried. For a woman who wanted to become pregnant, such a test can only be distressing. Testing kits containing two tests allow the woman to check her first result some time later or allows a second test to be carried out if a mistake has been made with the procedure in the first test.

11.2.2 Positive test results

For any pregnancy test which is performed in the pharmacy, if a positive result is obtained, then the woman must be strongly advised to make an appointment to see her doctor. This will ensure that appointments are made at an ante-natal clinic and that the woman is properly cared for during her pregnancy and also that she can be encouraged to make use of the health facilities available. Information about folic acid and encouragement to take it can also be offered. Some women will not wish to continue their pregnancy and, again, medical help must be sought. If the woman is reluctant to consult her family doctor, she could be referred to one of the pregnancy charities such as the British Pregnancy Advisory Service for medical advice.

11.2.3 Negative test results

If a woman's period is more than 5 days late but the pregnancy test produces a negative result, the advice to be given should be to see her GP. The reason for this is that there may be a serious reason for the negative test result, such as an ectopic pregnancy, which may sometimes cause a false-negative result.

11.2.4 Ovulation prediction kits

Once released, the ovum can live for between 12 and 24 hours. By having intercourse during this time, the couple will know that they are maximizing their chances of conception. The kits work by detecting a surge of luteinizing hormone (LH) which normally happens about 30 hours before the egg is released. The amount of time which elapses between the LH surge and ovulation may vary between 24 and 36 hours. The kits involve a daily test around the time that ovulation is expected. This would normally be around

14 days before the expected date of the next period, but even in women with regular cycles there may be a variation of 1 or 2 days either side of the expected time. For women who have irregular menstrual cycles, missing the LH surge can be a problem. The self-test ovulation kits may also fail to be effective if the LH surge is very brief and falls between the once-daily tests or if the level of LH is very low. Where the LH surge is thought to be brief, twice-daily testing will increase the chances of detection, but is a more expensive procedure. It may be better for the woman to learn fertility awareness methods.

A woman who wants to use a self-test kit but whose cycle is less regular can use a temperature chart method for a few months to establish the most likely days for ovulation. Women need to have 'normal' cycle lengths (not less than 23 days; not more than 35 days) to use this effectively.

Manufacturers of ovulation test kits recommend that any woman who does not conceive, or who fails to detect a surge of LH, after three menstrual cycles should go to see her GP for further discussions and investigations.

References

Centre for Pharmacy Postgraduate Education (1996) *Conception and Pregnancy*. University of Manchester.

Centre for Pharmacy Postgraduate Education (1997) *Contraception. A Distance Learning Package for Community Pharmacists*. University of Manchester.

The Family Planning Association (1999) *The Contraceptive Handbook*. fpa, 2–12 Pentonville Road, London N1 9FP.

Further help

fpa Information Service, for all information on contraception and sexual health, including publications for professionals and the public. Helpline 0171 837 4044; Library 0171 837 5228.

12 Women's health

The majority of community pharmacy customers are women. Pharmacists need to have an awareness of common conditions about which women may seek advice and treatment. The recurrence of many of these (for example vaginal thrush and cystitis) can be prevented or reduced by simple measures. This advice is at least as important as the treatment that can be offered. In addition, pharmacists need to know current thinking in osteoporosis prevention and treatment. In this chapter, we will consider some of the commonest conditions where the pharmacist's advice is likely to be sought and the practical advice that can be offered.

12.1 Cystitis

This is a common condition in which passing urine produces a painful burning sensation. The urge to pass urine occurs very frequently when, in fact, there is little to be voided. Although some cases of cystitis are due to bacterial infection (probably about half), a significant proportion have no apparent cause. Some women suffer from recurrent bouts and, although cystitis is classed by many as a minor condition, the level of discomfort and life disruption can be severe.

Intercourse itself may be a precipitating factor if damage to the urethra occurs, and 'honeymoon cystitis' is a well-known term. The irritant effect of soaps, bubble baths, and talcum powders can be a contributory factor in some women. Sensitivity reactions to rubber in condoms or constituents of other contraceptive products such as spermicides, caps, or diaphragms can also cause problems for some women. Simple advice about ensuring that the bladder is completely emptied can help. After the stream of urine has stopped, the woman should wait for about 30 seconds until after the last few drops have been passed. After passing a bowel motion, wiping from front to back with the toilet paper can prevent the transfer of bacteria into the vagina. Passing urine before and after intercourse can also help.

Over-the-counter treatments for cystitis are based on potassium or sodium citrate and they make the urine more alkaline. In cystitis, the urine becomes acidic and this is part of the reason why its passage is painful. Alkalinizing the urine reduces discomfort. Bacteria are less able to survive in alkaline urine, so this effect is also helpful.

A pregnant woman with cystitis should never be advised to try self-treatment for cystitis because untreated urinary tract infections in pregnancy can lead to serious kidney problems. Signs of such infection, such as fever, loin pain, and cloudy or smelly urine, would be indications for immediate referral to the GP rather than self-treatment.

As we have seen earlier, about half of the cases of cystitis are caused by a bacterial infection. The prescribing of antibiotics to treat urinary tract infections can result in vaginal thrush for some women. This is because the antibiotic wipes out the normal gut flora such that yeast infections are able to thrive. Antibiotics are generally not needed unless there are systemic signs of infection, as described above.

Where cystitis is a recurrent problem, self-help books such as Angela Kilmartin's *Understanding cystitis* are extremely valuable. Leaflets can also be helpful, and a recent study of a health education leaflet about cystitis showed that it reduced the number of subsequent consultations with the doctor. This suggests that more women need information about self-help measures in order for them to prevent future recurrences and to understand when it is important to see the GP rather than self-treat.

12.2   Vaginal thrush

Some women are prone to recurrent attacks of this infection, which often produces intense vaginal itching and a creamy white discharge. Predisposing factors include the use of broad-spectrum oral antibiotics which alter the balance of the body's usual bacterial flora and make conditions suitable for the yeast *Candida albicans* to grow. Warmth and moisture, increased by tight trousers, synthetic underwear, or leggings, are also common causes.

Pregnant women are more prone to vaginal thrush because of hormonal changes. Women with diabetes whose condition is not well controlled are prone to thrush because the sugar in their urine provides nutrients on which the yeast can feed. Unexplained recurrent attacks of thrush may be an early sign of diabetes. If the woman is experiencing weight loss, unusual and increasing thirst, and increasing passage of urine, she should be referred to her doctor immediately.

Treatment of vaginal thrush is straightforward as the most effective preparations can now be sold over the counter. There are two types of treatment—vaginal pessaries (clotrimazole and miconazole, for example) and an oral capsule (fluconazole). Both are effective and the choice of treatment should take into account the woman's preference. Over-the-counter thrush treatments cannot be used when a woman has not had thrush before. After the diagnosis of the first episode of thrush has been made by a doctor, future cases can be self-treated.

Self-help measures for thrush include the wearing of cotton (rather than nylon) underwear to allow the evaporation of perspiration. Wiping from front to back after passing a bowel motion can help to prevent the transmission of the yeast from the bowel to the vagina. The role of *Lactobacillus* in treating yeast infections has been the subject of debate for some years. The theoretical basis is that lactic acid is produced by the *Lactobacillus* and this will acidify the vaginal environment, making it more difficult for the yeast to grow. Some women do use yoghurt as a treatment (it needs to be 'live' yoghurt containing *Lactobacillus*) and apply it using a tampon.

12.3   Menstrual problems

It is estimated that one in two menstruating women suffer from dysmenorrhoea (period pains) and an even higher proportion from the pre-menstrual syndrome (PMS) in a mild to severe form.

Dysmenorrhoea can be treated with over-the-counter analgesics, of which ibuprofen is the most effective providing there are no contra-indications to its use. Pain at times of the cycle other than menstruation should be regarded with suspicion and requires referral.

PMS occurs when cyclical symptoms are experienced after ovulation in that part of the menstrual cycle which precedes the actual period. Such symptoms can be both physical (of which the commonest is breast tenderness) and emotional (including irritability and tiredness). Some studies have shown evening primrose oil to be effective in breast tenderness. Vitamin B6 (pyridoxine) at a dose of 10 mg a day has been shown to mitigate irritability, depression, and fatigue in PMS in some women. At the time of writing, there are proposals to restrict sales of pyridoxine to pharmacies at a daily dose of 50 mg or higher because of safety concerns. This is because of reported neurological side effects at very high doses in an early trial. There is no evidence of safety problems at lower doses.

12.4   Folic acid and neural tube defects

Research has shown that folic acid supplementation can reduce the incidence of neural tube defects such as spina bifida in babies. An educational campaign for women has followed and pharmacists have a number of opportunities to encourage folic acid use. Targeting women who are planning to have a child or have just found out they are pregnant are two obvious examples. The recommendation is that 400 mcg of folic acid is taken daily during the first three months of pregnancy, started before pregnancy if possible.

12.5   Menopausal problems

Research indicates that women's beliefs about the menopause are complex and that for many it is seen as a natural process that had to be 'gone through' by their mothers before them. The medicalization of the menopause is a relatively recent phenomenon, and women may be concerned about the use of unnatural substances (drugs) to treat a natural process. Resorting to treatment such as hormone replacement therapy (HRT) may be seen by the woman as a failure on her part.

A common problem for menopausal and post-menopausal women is vaginal dryness, which can make sexual intercourse uncomfortable and even painful. This is due to hormonal changes which result in natural vaginal lubrication being reduced through diminished oestrogen levels. Over-the-counter products are effective in the form of simple lubricants such as KY Jelly and the long-acting Replens. If such treatment is not successful, the woman should be referred to her doctor, who may prescribe an oestrogen vaginal cream which will correct the symptoms.

12.5.1 HRT

Pharmacists are sometimes asked by women about the effectiveness and safety of HRT following the menopause. Research shows that the majority of women have some awareness of HRT, mostly through the media. Many are also aware of the much-publicized potentially increased risk of breast cancer from HRT. The benefits of HRT include a protective effect against the development of osteoporosis and heart disease. The risks include a slight increase in the risk of breast cancer after long-term use. On a statistical basis, the woman is far more likely to suffer from osteoporosis or heart disease than from breast cancer. The pharmacist can offer information, and it is important that this is given in a neutral way to enable the woman to make her own decision. Research into HRT shows that the drop-out rate is high and that compliance is often poor. One possible reason for this may be that health professionals try to override womens' concerns, believing that they are doing the best thing by emphasizing the benefits of HRT.

HRT may be prescribed initially to help reduce severe symptoms associated with the menopause and with a longer-term intention of prevention of osteoporosis among women at risk. It is important that the woman understands where the treatment is intended to be continued and knows why this is proposed. The other key area of advice for pharmacists to give is to ensure that dietary intake of calcium and vitamin D is sufficient.

12.5.2 Osteoporosis

Osteoporosis is a condition which is common in elderly women (and to a lesser extent in men) and results from the loss of bone mass. The World Health Organization has drawn an analogy between osteoporosis, hypertension, and hypercholesterolaemia. All three are asymptomatic conditions until a major event of damage occurs. The risk of fractures occurring is greatly increased, and osteoporosis is estimated to be responsible for 150 000 fractures every year in the UK. Of these fractures, those of the hip have the most serious health consequences. Of every three patients with an osteoporotic hip fracture, one will die as a direct consequence. Another one of the three will require care in a nursing or residential home or other institution and will never be able to live independently again in their own home. The remaining one of the three is likely to lose some ability to perform normal daily tasks and thus will lose some of their independence. The problem of osteoporosis will become greater as the proportion of elderly people in the population rises. Causes include lack of physical exercise, smoking, excess alcohol, poor diet, and medication (notably long-term oral steroids).

The role of physical activity in preventing osteoporosis

Physical activity is the single most important measure in preventing both osteoporosis and the falls that are responsible for the fractures. Regular exercise should be started at as early an age as possible. In adulthood, exercise is of benefit in preserving bone density and may be important in maintaining bone strength. Even small percentages of bone mass and density preserved result in significant reductions in osteoporotic fractures. Regular physical activity also has beneficial protective effects on the heart and can be recommended for women of all ages. Swimming is an excellent form of aerobic exercise, with few contra-indications. Weight-bearing exercise such as brisk walking, climbing stairs, and dancing are of particular value. Among elderly people, strength and balance training are important and can reduce falls by a third (see Chapter 9, Physical activity).

The role of diet in osteoporosis

Calcium and vitamin D have an important role in maintaining healthy bone. Vitamin D is important in that it facilitates the absorption of calcium. In addition to its direct involvement in bone formation, calcium may also increase the beneficial effect of HRT and perhaps calcitonin on bone mineral density. The key advice for pharmacists to give is to ensure that dietary intake of calcium and vitamin D is sufficient. For women aged 19 and over, the daily reference nutrient intake (RNI) is 700 mg.

Dietary sources of calcium

Milk, half pint (skimmed, semi-skimmed, whole) 350 mg

Yoghurt (150 g carton) 250–300 mg

Cheddar cheese 360 mg

Sardines, canned (70 g) 350 mg

Green vegetables, (100 g) 50–150 mg

Beans/lentils, (100 g) 100 mg

The possible role of supplementation is more complex, but calcium supplementation should be considered in the elderly and in adolescents where the dietary intake seems to be inadequate.

In post-menopausal women, calcium supplements may help to slow the rate of bone loss but cannot prevent it. Research findings indicate that this effect may become more important 5 years and more after the menopause. In pre-menopausal women, some studies have shown a beneficial effect of calcium on bone mineral density while others have not.

The ability to absorb vitamin D from dietary sources may decrease with age, and elderly people are at particular risk of deficiency of this vitamin.

12.6   Case studies

1. *A woman presents a prescription for HRT patches. It is the first time you have dispensed this for her and your pharmacy policy on first dispensing is to ask whether the patient has had the preparation before. In response to your question, she tells you that her GP has just prescribed it. She goes on to say that she went to the GP mainly for reassurance. She is going through the menopause and has recently felt like she wanted to 'explode' with irritation and anger. Her husband was keen for her to 'get it sorted out'. When you ask how she feels about using HRT she says she doesn't really want to use it.*

Here the pharmacist needs to find out what this woman already knows about HRT, including what the doctor has said about how long the treatment is intended for. She is already expressing doubts about using HRT and it is important that she has the opportunity to express her concerns. The reality is that women do decide to stop using HRT, or to use it less frequently than prescribed, without telling the doctor or pharmacist. Enabling an open discussion may help, and in the informal atmosphere of the pharmacy women may feel more comfortable to voice their real thoughts. As part of the discussion, the pharmacist can provide up to date information on the benefits and risks of HRT. Going through the manufacturer's information leaflet can be useful, recognizing that these tend to include more about risks than about benefits of treatment. The pharmacist's goal should not be to try to persuade this woman to use HRT if this is not what she wants. However, it is the pharmacist's goal to help her to reach an informed decision. She may want to take the information away with her and make her decision later.

2. *A woman asks for advice about osteoporosis. Her mother who is 65 fell last week and broke her wrist. At the hospital, a DEXA scan diagnosed osteoporosis.*

The pharmacist can check if this woman's mother is taking any regular medication and if so whether this might have contributed to the fall. If the pharmacist suspects that this might be the case, the GP should be contacted to discuss the treatment. Next the pharmacist can enquire about diet. Elderly people may need supplements of calcium and vitamin D depending on dietary intake and access to sunlight (housebound people, for example, have less exposure to sunlight and this may be a cause of vitamin D deficiency). Enquiring about physical activity is also important. Building strength and balance can help to prevent future falls. The pharmacist might recommend contacting the local Age Concern branch or other group to find out what sorts of exercise classes are arranged for older people. Even frail elderly people can participate in and benefit from appropriate exercise.

13 Baby and child health

Mothers of young children are a major group of pharmacy customers and will ask the pharmacist about many aspects of baby and child health. Often such queries will relate to specific symptoms, but in many cases it is general health advice and an intelligent interpretation of current evidence that is needed. In the past, young mothers would have obtained much of their advice and guidance from their own mothers. Now that families are often geographically distant, there may be a greater need for advice from pharmacists, health visitors, and GPs.

There are four main areas for advice:

1. Practical aspects, e.g. infant feeding
2. Common and recurrent public health problems, e.g. head lice, threadworms
3. Topical issues, e.g. the latest research on child nutrition
4. Common misconceptions, e.g. that antibiotics are always needed in infections

Practical advice is often needed about routine aspects of caring for a baby such as feeding choice and practice, and for the treatment of common problems such as nappy rash, where the pharmacist can also offer advice about preventing recurrence. Awareness of current practice is essential to reflect current thinking on issues such as when to introduce solids and cow's milk into the baby's diet.

Some problems are seasonal and regular, for example an epidemic of head lice at the local school, when the pharmacist must know the current advice on the use of insecticides and on 'bug-busting' policies.

Other problems will be prompted by media publicity. A recurrent example is the sensational reports of brain damage caused by whooping cough vaccination, where what is needed from the pharmacist is an informed analysis of the risks and benefits. For such issues of topical concern, the pharmacist is able to give the facts, where these are clearly known, or to make an appraisal of the evidence to date, and to err on the side of caution where there is any doubt.

Correcting widespread and deeply held misconceptions is another important area for pharmacists' advice, for example the idea that antibiotic therapy is always needed in the treatment of infections. Concerned parents may seek advice from the pharmacist about their child's prescription, and a clear explanation together with reassurance are needed.

13.1   Vaccination and immunization

While vaccination may not generate many direct inquiries to the pharmacist, it is nevertheless essential that the pharmacist is aware of current vaccination schedules and knows the rationale behind each in order to respond should queries arise. With the increasing emphasis on preventive care and the requirement to reach set targets in the GP contract, parents will be contacted to ensure their children are vaccinated. Pharmacies are an obvious place to display leaflets on vaccination, and these may generate questions in the informal atmosphere of the pharmacy. Indeed, the pharmacist may take a more pro-active role, offering such leaflets when dispensing prescriptions for babies and young children. The current vaccination schedule is shown below.

1. In the first year of life, three doses of diphtheria, pertussis, tetanus, polio, and *Haemophilus influenzae* type b vaccines. The first is given at 2 months of age, the second at 3 months, and the third at 4 months.

2. In the second year of life, the measles, mumps, and rubella vaccine (MMR) is given, generally between 12 and 15 months.

3. At school entry, or entry to nursery school, MMR, diphtheria, tetanus, and polio vaccine boosters are given.

4. Between the tenth and fourteenth birthdays, the BCG vaccine is given for tuberculin-negative children.

13.1.1   Pertussis (whooping cough)

Some 10 000 cases of pertussis were notified in 1989. Following many media reports of brain damage caused by pertussis vaccine, the percentage of infants who were vaccinated fell drastically during the 1970s. While the link between pertussis vaccine and brain damage is contentious and still provokes much debate, there is no doubt that the disease itself can cause brain damage. Estimates are that 1 in 500 cases of whooping cough result in brain damage, and the disease can be fatal. For the vaccine, epidemiological studies estimate that 1 in 100 000 injections resulted in a neurological reaction, most of which involved prolonged febrile convulsions from which most infants recovered without adverse consequences.

13.1.2   Measles, mumps and rubella (MMR)

The combined measles, mumps, and rubella vaccine was introduced in October 1988 with the aim of eliminating congenital rubella syndrome, measles, and mumps. While many people consider rubella, measles, and mumps to be 'harmless' diseases of childhood, this is far from the case. Measles has serious complications including encephalitis, which can be fatal. In adults, mumps can cause orchitis (inflammation of the testes) in males and even sterility. Congenital rubella syndrome results where damage is done to the developing fetus when the mother becomes infected with rubella (German measles) during pregnancy. Multiple congenital defects including heart problems, deafness, and cataracts may result.

After-effects following MMR include malaise, fever, and rash, usually about a week after injection. Swelling of the parotid glands (those which are affected by mumps) can also occur at a later stage of around 3 weeks after vaccination.

In 1998, there was concern about a possible association between MMR vaccination and cases of autism. A detailed analysis of the evidence found no association between the two.

13.1.3   Contra-indications to vaccination

Contra-indications to vaccination is an area where there is much misunderstanding among both health professionals and members of the public. Vaccination should be postponed if the child is suffering from a febrile illness because the body's immune system is already activated and may destroy the vaccine before antibodies are made.

Minor infections without fever or systemic upset are not contra-indications.

It is widely believed by members of the public and others that children who suffer from eczema or other allergic conditions should not receive vaccinations. This is not the case. The *British National Formulary* sets out advice on contra-indications for each vaccine and advises that the doctor should seek specialist advice from the local paediatrics department before deciding not to vaccinate a child.

13.1.4   Paracetamol in feverish reactions

Paracetamol syrup can be given, together with tepid sponging to reduce the temperature. Parents need to know that sponging with cold water can cause a further rise in temperature by shutting down blood vessels close to the skin surface, thereby reducing heat loss through the skin. Tepid water should therefore be used. Pharmacists may be asked if paracetamol can be given to infants under 3 months who become feverish following the first dose of diphtheria, pertussis, and polio vaccination. The *British National Formulary* recommends a dose of 5–10 mg/kg on the advice of a doctor. Guidelines are that for 2-month-old full-term infants 60 mg should be given, and that for 2-month-old pre-term infants 10 mg/kg should be given. The small doses involved mean that oral syringes will be required to measure accurately.

13.2   Infant feeding

Most mothers will seek advice from the health visitor or baby clinic about feeding, and this advice will be of a high standard. Advice is also sought from pharmacists and, while it is appropriate for pharmacists to encourage breastfeeding and to give advice which will support this, it is not the pharmacist's role to suggest that a baby is fed with formula milk. Thus if the mother is experiencing difficulties in breastfeeding she should be referred to her health visitor, GP, or baby clinic to discuss the problems being encountered. If a formula feed is required, advice will then be given about its selection. Where a mother has been advised by the health visitor to use a formula feed or has decided independently to do so, then it would be appropriate for the pharmacist to offer advice about the selection of a product and its correct use.

13.2.1   Breastfeeding

Expert opinion is agreed that breastfeeding is best for all babies and confers several benefits. Research has shown clearly that breast-feeding, even if only for a period of 12 weeks, will give the baby protection against a variety of infections, particularly those of the respiratory tract. Almost all formula feeds are modified cow's milk and, whilst technical developments have meant that the nutritional composition of milk has been made to closely resemble that of breast milk, the nature of the protein is different. Breast milk is the more easily digestible and is always preferable to formula milks.

The *British National Formulary* summarizes those drugs which, when taken by the mother, are transferred into breast milk. The relevant section is 'Prescribing during breastfeeding'. Over-the-counter medicines need to be considered as well as prescribed medicines. There has been publicity about the possible effects of coffee drinking by breastfeeding mothers. Young babies are known to metabolize caffeine more slowly than adults, and irritability in a baby whose mother consumes a lot of tea or coffee may be helped by a switch to decaffeinated versions. Fizzy drinks such as cola can be high in caffeine, so caffeine-free varieties are to be preferred.

Mothers may sometimes ask for advice about breastfeeding, and the pharmacy should stock a range of the accessories and equip-ment to facilitate this. When the baby feeds at one breast, milk leaks from the other, and breast shells made of moulded plastic can be worn to collect the drips of milk. They should be sterilized before use. Breast pads are worn to catch drops of milk. They can be worn continuously to prevent wetting of clothes and are available in disposable and washable versions. A breast pump can be used to express milk which can then be stored in the fridge; the milk can also be frozen so long as it is used within 4 weeks. Nipple shields protect the skin, and creams are available for sore or cracked nipples. If the nipples are very painful, the woman needs to be referred to her GP as infection (mastitis) may have occurred.

13.2.2 Bottle feeding

The range of baby milks on the pharmacy shelf is extensive. Whey-based milks have formulae which are closest to breast milk and are most easily digested by the baby. Curd-based milks contain a higher proportion of curd protein (casein) and are said to be more satisfying for hungrier babies. This is because the curds stay in the stomach for longer and take longer to digest, giving a feeling of fullness. Other formula milks include those which are soya-based and suitable for babies who are allergic to cow's milk. Symptoms of such an allergy include crying after feeds, vomiting, and diarrhoea. Fortunately, most babies grow out of their allergy by the age of 2 years. Pharmacists should not, however, recommend a switch to soya-based milk and it is better to advise the mother to seek advice from her health visitor or the GP.

Low-lactose feeds are designed to be given following a bout of gastroenteritis, when a temporary lactose intolerance is not uncommon. After the first 6 months of life, 'follow on' milks are available which are given until the end of the first year.

A good policy is to become familiar with one or two product ranges and to get up to date literature from the company representatives about new research and developments. Remember always to include a verbal reinforcement of the manufacturer's written advice about hygiene and sterilization of bottles and teats, and about the transmission of infection via inadequately cleaned feeding equipment.

13.2.3 Cow's milk and babies

Cow's milk should not be introduced into the baby's diet before the age of 1 year. Because of the growing baby's need for calories, semi-skimmed should not be given below the age of 2 years and skimmed milk not below 5 years. Semi-skimmed and skimmed milks should only be given to children of the appropriate ages if their diet is satisfactory in terms of calorie and nutrient intake.

13.2.4 Crying and colic

Babies have been observed to cry characteristically and draw up their legs in the early evenings after feeds up to the age of 3 months. Such crying was thought to be due to colic ('three month colic') and babies were given gripe water and other remedies. Research now suggests that the crying pattern has no connection with symptoms and that, while early evening crying does reach a peak between the ages of 2 and 3 months, there was no evidence of symptoms in most babies. Some infants undoubtedly suffer from wind and, while simethicone or dimethicone were traditionally recommended, a more recent analysis of research findings has not shown them to be effective in colic. The same analysis of research indicated that a trial of different milk might be appropriate in bottle-fed babies, together with referral to the health visitor for further advice.

Pharmacists need to bear in mind the stress which is caused to parents by a crying baby and try to reassure them that crying is not always caused by hunger pangs. The parents also need to listen for unusual kinds of crying and to be reminded that crying babies can often be pacified by cuddling, speaking, and singing, as well as by feeding.

13.2.5 Drinks between feeds

Boiled, cooled water (unsweetened) can be given or one of the ranges of baby drinks and fruit juices. Careful label watching is required to find low-sugar varieties.

13.2.6 Weaning

Between the ages of 4 and 6 months, babies are generally ready to move on to solid foods in addition to their milk. Weaning should not take place before 4 months, because evidence from research suggests that early weaning may result in a greater likelihood of allergies. Some experts suggest that rice is a good weaning food rather than wheat-based cereals, and all weaning foods should be gluten-free.

13.2.7 Diarrhoea and vomiting

Rehydration therapy is the only treatment recommended for diarrhoea and vomiting in infants and young children. The risks of dehydration mean that fluid and electrolyte intake are critical. Babies aged under 1 year who have diarrhoea and vomiting should always be referred to the GP, although rehydration therapy can be started. For children over 1 year, referral is advisable if the condition continues for longer than 24 hours or worsens in the meantime. Again, rehydration sachets should be recommended.

13.2.8 Responding to symptoms in babies

Some pharmacist experts argue that it is not appropriate to recommend medicines for use in babies under 1 year old. Bearing in mind the possible hazards of doing so (for example rapid dehydration occurring in infections and diarrhoea; abdominal pain of unknown cause; changes in crying pattern; and so on), the possible complications and difficulty in establishing the cause of some symptoms mean that great care should be exercised by pharmacists and their staff.

13.2.9 Vitamin supplements

Babies from the age of 6 months to 2 years who are not receiving breast or formula milk, and preferably up to 5 years old, should receive multivitamin supplements. Mothers attending a baby clinic will be advised about vitamin supplementation. Vitamin drops can be bought at Well Baby clinics at a reduced price. Mothers who visit the pharmacy can be asked whether vitamin drops are being given. If not, they can be obtained either from the baby clinic, on prescription from the GP, or purchased over the counter.

For older children, parents are often concerned at what they consider to be faddy eating habits and think that their children may be vitamin deficient. Hence they may ask pharmacists for suitable vitamin products. The pharmacist can encourage the keeping of a food diary to assess what is actually eaten by the child so that recommendations can be made about important foods to be added. The pharmacist can also enquire about the child's weight and general development to ascertain whether these are within normal limits. If the child is seriously underweight, they will need more than just vitamins. Very often it is the case that parents are needlessly anxious about the tension which is associated with mealtimes with a child who refuses to eat particular foods. In addition, television and magazine advertising tend to suggest that all children will benefit from vitamin supplementation.

There have been claims that multivitamin and mineral supplements can improve the IQ of children. On current evidence, routine supplementation for children cannot be recommended. However, if the food diary indicates that low amounts of particular vitamins are being taken in the diet, supplementation should be considered if attempts to encourage the child to eat certain foods are not successful. Further studies are being carried out to provide data on vitamin and mineral supplementation and intelligence.

13.3   General dietary advice

The general advice on healthy eating outlined in Chapter 8 should not be followed in its entirety for young children. While there is evidence that children receive more saturated fat than is ideal, and this should be reduced, it is not recommended that children receive a large quantity of fibre. The danger is that, in their smaller gut, the increased fibre is likely to lead to a reduced appetite, with the possibility that they will not eat sufficient food to prevent malnourishment. In addition, fibre can reduce the absorption of some vitamins. Experts are generally agreed that for children of 12 and under, a sensible approach would be gradually to reduce the calories obtained from fat between the ages of 2 and 5. Fibre can be increased gradually and slowly from this age. The best guide is weight and general fitness. Underweight children may have serious eating problems, but they may also have too much fibre in their diet, so that they become full too quickly and are not taking in sufficent calories. Overweight children should not be given sweet snacks between meals and their diet should be adjusted to include less sugar and fat.

13.3.1   Sugar and dental caries

Wherever possible in responding to symptoms in children, the pharmacist should recommend a sugar-free medicine. Such formulations are now available for most therapeutic uses. Many pharmacies stock and sell items of confectionery, for example barley sugars and other sweets. The RPSGB's Code of Ethics states that items of confectionery should not be placed at or near the till or in easy reach of small children. The sale of sweets is difficult to reconcile with a health promotion role, especially one in which advice on oral health from the pharmacist is increasingly recognized.

From the weaning stage, parents should not add sugar and salt to food. If sweets are to be given to children, they are best eaten immediately after a meal, and the teeth brushed afterwards. Babies and children who wake during the night should be given water (boiled and cooled first in the case of babies).

13.4　Head lice

Pharmacists commonly are asked to recommend prevention and treatment for head lice. Given concerns about possible resistance to insecticides, treatment should only be used where live lice have been found. The best approach is therefore to encourage regular examination of the child's hair and the pharmacist can explain how to do this. Head lice are spread through head to head contact and, because the symptoms do not become apparent until after several hundred lice bites, other family members may have been infected. The long association between poor hygiene and head lice is totally inaccurate. Despite the commonness of lice infection, many parents still feel that there is a stigma and are embarrassed that their child has got lice. Pharmacists need to bear in mind that customers asking for treatment or information about head lice may feel ashamed and embarrassed. Suggesting a move to a quieter area of the pharmacy may be welcomed. Pharmacists should not belittle customers' concerns by making humorous comments in an attempt to set someone at their ease. Instead, the pharmacist needs to be sensitive, picking up on verbal and non-verbal signals to respond.

The old district treatment rotation policy approach is now not carried out in many areas. Instead, mosaic treatment, where one client is recommended a particular insecticide, the next a different one, and so on, is increasingly used. 'Bug-buster' programmes where the use of repeat combing is the only treatment appear to be gaining in popularity.

The main insecticides used are malathion, permethrin (available over the counter), and carbaryl (Prescription Only status). Shampoo formulations of malathion and carbaryl are no longer considered effective and should not be recommended. The potential problem with treatment is that not only the live lice but also the eggs must be killed. It is important to follow the manufacturers' instructions for treatment.

Both carbaryl and malathion are inactivated by heat, and parents should be advised that the hair should be left to dry naturally after applying the lotion rather than using a hair dryer or sitting close to a heat source. Both insecticides are also inactivated by chlorine in swimming pools and, if the child has been swimming before treatment, the hair should be shampooed thoroughly before applying the insecticide.

Parents are sometimes confused that after treatment the empty egg shells or 'nits' can still be seen in the hair and think this means the treatment has not worked. The nits are firmly glued to the hair and will not be removed simply by shampooing. The use of a fine toothcomb can be recommended and, to make the process more comfortable, the hair should be combed after applying conditioner (any sort will do) so that the comb runs through the hair more readily.

Treatment failure is generally because the product has not been used properly or, more probably, because the child's head has become reinfected by a family member or at school. School staff sometimes make recommendations about head lice treatment, and pharmacists can ensure that they have the most current information.

Parents are rightly concerned about the safety issues associated with insecticides, especially in repeated use. In some areas, head lice reinfection after treatment is common and parents worry that their child might have numerous doses of insecticide. The current evidence does not indicate that use of insecticides on the scalp to treat head lice is likely to lead to adverse effects. However, parents' concerns need to be taken seriously. If a parent wants to try the combing method rather than use an insecticide, this decision should be respected.

13.5   Threadworms

Like head lice, the subject of threadworm infection is the cause of much anxiety and distress, both to children and to their parents. It has been estimated that, at any one time, between 20 and 30 per cent of schoolchildren aged under 10 years will be infected with threadworms. This infection is a common problem which rarely needs medical treatment and can be dealt with effectively by treatment and advice from the pharmacist. The characteristic appearance of these worms led to their name, and the worms resemble small threads of white cotton. They can be seen in the faeces or around the anus. The infection is transferred by eggs which are found commonly under the fingernails. The eggs are swallowed after finger sucking or nail biting and then move into the gastrointestinal tract, finally hatching in the lower portion of the large bowel. At night, the female worms emerge to lay eggs on the perianal skin, and these eggs are secreted in a sticky, glue-like substance which is responsible for the symptomatic itch. The skin is scratched, more eggs are transferred under the fingernails and the whole process begins again.

Mebendazole is now the most recommended treatment. Parents need to be aware that while treatment will kill the existing worms, other action is also needed to break the cycle of infection. Advice should include keeping the fingernails short, wearing of pyjamas in bed, having a warm bath after getting up in the morning (this helps to wash away the newly laid eggs from the night before), and thorough cleaning of the nails using a nail brush. It is generally recommended that all family members are treated at the same time, since symptoms may not manifest themselves for some time after the initial infection has taken place.

13.6   Bedwetting

Parents sometimes ask pharmacists for advice and treatment for bedwetting (nocturnal enuresis). The pharmacist should be aware of the normal pattern and development of bladder control in children and of the reassuring statistics that can be offered to worried parents. One large study found that 1 in 20 children aged 7 wet the bed at least once a week; by the age of 10, only one in 40 do so. Bedwetting is commoner among boys than girls. Recent life changes such as starting school or being in hospital can induce enuresis in a child who has become dry. Pharmacists should be alert for symptoms of urinary tract infections which may sometimes precipitate a problem of bedwetting.

There is a variety of mechanical aids and alarms which are intended to awaken the child as soon as the first drops of urine are passed in order to prompt him to go to the toilet. These devices have become increasingly sophisticated and acceptable to parent and child. Child psychologists who have dealt with the problem of bedwetting are agreed that a system of small rewards is an effective means of encouraging 'dryness', whereas disapproval and punishments have the opposite to the desired effect.

A medical referral should be made, since further investigations and drug treatment may need to be initiated. Medical referral should also be advised if the pharmacist suspects that a urinary tract infection may be the cause of the problem. Some school nurses have bed alarms which can be loaned for a 3-month trial period via the GP, who monitors progress. The pharmacist could find out which of the local schools have this facility.

13.7 Childhood infections and antibiotics

Parents sometimes expect the GP to prescribe antibiotics for a child who has an upper respiratory tract or ear infection. However, evidence does not support such prescribing, and concerns about antimicrobial resistance resulted in key government reports recommending reduced prescribing of antibiotics. Research findings suggest that expectation of prescribed antibiotics is a learned behaviour and that when they are prescribed for respiratory tract infections the patient is more likely to consult their doctor about the same symptoms in the future.

Parents may complain to the pharmacist that their child has not received the treatment he or she needs. There is an important role for the pharmacist in explaining the difference between viral and bacterial infections in simple terms and explaining why antibiotics do not work in viral infections.

13.8   Case studies

1. 'I've had a letter about vaccinations—but they can be dangerous can't they?'

A young mother who was a regular customer asked this question in response to the pharmacist's enquiry about the health of her recently born baby. The baby is now 3 months old and should have had his first diphtheria, pertussis, polio, and HIb vaccine last month. The pharmacist asked 'What makes you think that vaccinations are dangerous?' and the woman replied that she had heard about babies having brain damage afterwards. Giving the woman a leaflet about infant vaccinations, the pharmacist explained that there appeared to be a very small chance of brain damage from the whooping cough element of the vaccine. However, she went on, the modern vaccine is very highly purified and less likely to cause such problems. She also said it was important to be aware that whooping cough itself can have very serious consequences, and that the chance of these occurring was higher than of serious problems as a result of the vaccine. The pharmacist suggested that the woman might want to talk to her GP or health visitor before making a final decision.

2. 'There's nits going around at the school. My children haven't got them but what can I use to make sure they don't?'

The pharmacist's heart sank on hearing this question—a common one and often a difficult explanation to get across. She explained that the treatments available for head lice did not work in preventing them and that if they were used when they were not needed they may not work so well in the future. She asked the woman if she would know what to look for if checking whether lice were present and explained how to examine the hair and use combing over a light coloured surface to detect lice. When examining the hair she advised paying particular attention to the nape of the neck, under the fringe, and behind the ears. If a child was infected, empty egg shells (nits) would be seen, white or greyish in colour. Tiny eggs might also be seen closer to the hair roots and waiting to hatch out. These, however, would be more difficult to spot. A treatment would then be needed.

The woman was not convinced. Wasn't there anything she could buy, she asked? The pharmacist explained that one product was available that claimed to repel lice. It worked, she said, by making the hair feel cooler and, as lice preferred warm scalps, the theory was they should be put off by this. She also suggested that the woman might comb the childrens' hair with a fine-toothed comb after applying conditioner.

3. *'My baby's got an awful cough and the doctor's just been, but he wouldn't give her any antibiotics. It's not very good, is it? Do you think these young doctors know enough?'*

This young mother was worried about her young child's cough and believed that antibiotics were the correct treatment. This was largely because the previous doctor had always prescribed them for her other children when they were young. The pharmacist asked her what the doctor had said. She remembered that he had examined the baby, listened to her chest, and said something about a virus. The pharmacist briefly explained about the different sorts of infections and how research had shown that antibiotics did not improve most coughs because the vast majority are caused by viruses. She also explained the worries about antibiotics being used too much and that they might not work properly in the future. She went on to say that because the doctor had examined the child, he had made sure that antibiotics were not needed. Finally, she suggested some practical measures like using steam in the bedroom to humidify the air (by boiling a kettle for 10–15 minutes in there before the baby was put to bed) and suggested that a soothing mixture such as Paediatric Simple Linctus may also help.

14 Travel health

An increasing number of pharmacy customers are travelling to remote parts of the world for both pleasure and business. Younger travellers have a higher risk of illness. The greater the climatic and cultural differences between the traveller's country of origin and destination, the greater the risk of illness. Pharmacists are well placed to give advice about staying healthy abroad including immunization, malaria prophylaxis, safety, and hygiene, as well as use of sunscreens and treatment of diarrhoea. In this chapter, we also discuss skin cancer and its prevention, an area where pharmacists have a unique role to play in advising on sun protection.

Pharmacists should keep and display information leaflets about staying healthy abroad. These leaflets often contain checklists for the traveller to ensure that they have made all necessary purchases. The pharmacist's first contact with someone who is travelling is often when they ask for antimalarials. This should be taken as a cue to advise them about immunizations, insect repellents, sun protection, and so on.

14.1 Malaria prophylaxis

Malaria is the single most important hazard facing travellers to tropical countries and is largely preventable if appropriate precautions are taken. Malaria is a parasitic disease spread by *Anopheles* mosquitoes; between 200 and 300 million people are affected by the disease each year. About 2000 people returning to the UK after travel each year have become infected with malaria. The most important way of reducing the risk of malaria is to reduce the number of insect bites by using insect repellents of which DEET (diethyl toluamide) is probably the most widely used. DEET is available in the UK in a range of formulations including sprays, gels, and lotions. The most important points of advice are to use a preparation with a concentration of 30–50 per cent, and to reapply every 4 hours. DEET can be applied to the skin, clothing, or wrist and ankle bands, especially in the evening and when out of doors at night. Travellers should also be told to wear long trousers and long sleeves at night.

Further protection while sleeping can be obtained by using a mosquito net impregnated with permethrin insecticide; air conditioning, if available, reduces the chance of being bitten. Pharmacists can also sell electric mosquito killers in which tablets containing pyrethroids are placed. *Anopheles* mosquitoes prefer to bite between dusk and dawn, so it is important to be vigilant at this time.

Advice about which antimalarials to recommend for which country is found in the latest editions of the *British National Formulary*, *MIMS*, and in National Pharmaceutical Association updates. The print versions are updated approximately every 6 months, and *British National Formulary* section 5.4 gives a list of telephone numbers for obtaining advice about specific problems. The advice is that of UK experts, for residents of the UK, who travel to endemic areas for short stays. The choice of drugs takes into account the risk of exposure to malaria, the extent of drug resistance, efficacy of the recommended drugs, side-effects of the drugs, and patient-related criteria such as age, pregnancy, epilepsy, and renal or hepatic function. Where a journey requires two or more regimens, the regimen for the higher risk area should be used for the whole journey. Settled immigrants (or long-term visitors) to the UK may be unaware that they well have lost their immunity to malaria and also that the area where they previously lived may now be malarious. It is important that pharmacists working in areas with minority ethnic groups put this message across.

Chemoprophylaxis should be started 1 week before departure (3 weeks for mefloquine), but not later than the first day of exposure, and be continued for at least 4 weeks after return. All tablets should be taken with or after food, or nausea can occur, especially with chloroquine. Travellers should also be advised to be extra vigilant about covering up and using insect repellents if they are suffering from diarrhoea or vomiting, as they then may not fully absorb their antimalarial tablets.

Pregnant women should avoid travelling to malarious areas because prophylaxis is not completely effective and a woman's resistance to malaria falls. Malaria tends to be more severe in pregnancy and there is an increased risk of prematurity, miscarriage, and stillbirth. However, the benefits of prophylaxis outweigh the risks, and if pregnant women have to travel to endemic regions they should take proguanil and chloroquine because the other medicines have teratogenic potential. If they are taking folic acid for the prevention of neural tube defects and are also taking proguanil, they should increase their dose of folic acid to 5 mg daily. Pregnant women who are taking proguanil should also be advised to take folic acid. Pharmacists are not allowed to sell more than a 500 mcg dose, so should refer pregnant women to their GP for a prescription. Breast-fed infants should receive prophylaxis as although antimalarials are excreted in breast milk, the amounts are too variable to give reliable protection.

Pharmacists should warn travellers that they should report any flu-like illness to their GP for up to a year and especially within 3 months of returning form an endemic area, as it is possible that they might have malaria, even if all precautions have been taken.

14.2   Immunization

Pharmacists may be called upon to give advice about immunization for travellers. They may also use other opportunities such as when someone asks about malaria prophylaxis to ensure that the person has been immunized. No particular immunization is required for travellers to Europe, the United States, Australia, or new Zealand, although all travellers should have immunity to tetanus and poliomyelitis (childhood immunizations should be up to date). In non-European areas surrounding the Mediterranean, Africa, South and Central America, and Asia, certain special precautions are required. The *British National Formulary* contains up to date advice for travellers, and pharmacists should refer people to their GP or to a travel clinic for advice and immunizations.

14.3   Traveller's diarrhoea

Diarrhoea is by far the most common problem affecting travellers. Up to 50 per cent of all travellers suffer at some stage. At least

80 per cent of traveller's diarrhoea is caused by infections. Most episodes are short lived; any episode that continues for longer than 72 hours and/or continues on return to the UK should be referred to the GP, as should any episode of diarrhoea involving blood in the stools. Most cases are caused by microorganisms including bacteria, viruses, and protozoa. Travellers should be told to take a number of precautions to avoid contracting diarrhoea, most cases being caused by swallowing contaminated material. Travellers must avoid food and drink that has a high risk of being contaminated and if they have to eat with their fingers (expected in some cultures) they should ensure that they are scrupulously clean and dry. In practice, freshly and well-cooked food is usually safe; avoid reheated food, salads, unpasteurized milk, and ice lollies and ice cream, and always peel fruit.

Travellers should avoid drinking local tap water, choosing bottled water instead. Carbonated drinks which are also acidic are usually safe. Fizzy drinks are also more difficult to counterfeit. Ice is as safe as the water from which it is made and should usually be avoided. Those travelling to more remote areas where bottled water cannot be obtained or carried should sterilize any water by boiling then filtering with special filters (probably best) or chemically treating it with, for example, iodine or chlorine. Pharmacists may be asked to supply iodine or water purification tablets for this purpose.

Travellers diarrhoea is commonly caused by *E.coli*. *Shigella* (bacterial dysentery), *Salmonella* and rotaviruses can also cause it, as can *Giardia* and *Entaemoba histolytica* (amoebic dysentery).

Travellers should be given practical advice about how to treat acute diarrhoea. Those with severe or prolonged diarrhoea should seek medical advice rather than self-medicate. Those travelling to remote areas are often advised to take antibiotics with them to self-treat if necessary. The general advice is to carry the antibiotics because of supply problems, but to try to find a doctor if at all possible.

There remains a reluctance among health professionals to recommend anything for diarrhoea other than oral rehydration therapy, even for adults. This is largely due to a belief that antimotility drugs will prolong or worsen an infection. This is not supported by the evidence for the majority of causes of diarrhoea.

Antidiarrhoeals such as loperamide are probably the first line treatment in adults. Loperamide increases the tone of both the small and large bowel and reduces intestinal motility. It also increases sphincter tone and decreases intestinal secretary activity. Decreased motility enhances fluid and electrolyte reabsorption and decreases the volume of the intestinal contents, aiding reabsorption of water. A recent study showed that loperamide produced complete relief from diarrhoea in a median time of 25 hours, compared with 40 hours for placebo. Antidiarrhoeals may cause problems if used in diarrhoea due to dysentery; however, only 5 per cent of cases of traveller's diarrhoea are due to this. Antidiarrhoeals can also cause constipation. Rehydration should still be emphasized as well as the anti-diarrhoeal.

Oral rehydration therapy should be used for children and can be used by adults as well, especially in tropical climates where risk of dehydration is greatest. Travellers should be reminded never to make up the sachets with local tap water.

14.4   Diabetics and travel

Pharmacists may be asked for advice by diabetic travellers. The British Diabetic Association produce an excellent leaflet that pharmacists can make available.

Journeys across time zones may mean that insulin-dependent diabetics have to adjust their insulin. When travelling from east to west, the day is lengthened and some clinics advise diabetics to take an extra meal to cover it. Special airline meals for diabetics are often very low in carbohydrate, and it is better for diabetics to order the standard meal. In general, if the time zone is changing by less than 4 hours, diabetics will not need to change their insulin injections. Any changes in insulin dosing should be discussed with the patient's diabetic team prior to departure,

Many people now have three short-acting injections a day and a medium- or long-acting injection in the evening; this can easily be adapted with time zone travel. If diabetics travel regularly, they are usually switched to this system. Those who take tablets for their diabetes are unlikely to have any problems. Very occasionally they may be advised to take an additional tablet to cover long days or to

leave out a dose on short days (a long west to east journey).
Diabetics should always carry glucose tablets and carbohydrate
food with them. On long journeys, they should check their blood
glucose before and after the journey and two or three times on the
plane.

14.5   Sunscreens and skin cancer

Exposure to sunlight prematurely ages the skin and brings the risk
of skin cancer.

Sun protection is a crucial part of skin cancer prevention
strategies and pharmacies are an ideal place to promote it.
Pharmacists can offer advice on the use of sunscreens and other
protective measures.

Those most at risk of skin cancer are fair-skinned, fair or red-
haired, with light-coloured eyes, who never tan or who burn before
they tan. Also at risk are those with a large number of ordinary
moles (over 60 in young people, over 50 in older people). Unusual
moles which change shape (large, irregular, and multi-coloured) are
a risk factor. Another risk factor is a family history of melanoma,
or having previously had a melanoma.

14.5.1   Sun protection

Sunscreens are classified according to their sun protection factor
(SPF). This is the ratio of the minimal dose of UVB radiation
necessary to produce delayed erythema in skin protected by the
sunscreen to that in unprotected skin. The higher the SPF, the
greater protection afforded to the skin. The classification of skin
types is shown in Table 14.1.

The Imperial Cancer Research Fund (ICRF) give the following
tips to parents to enable children to enjoy the summer safely.

1. Keep children out of the sun when it is at its most dangerous—
   between 11 a.m. and 3 p.m. Carers of young children should
   make every effort to schedule their outdoor activities to avoid
   this time of day.

Table 14.1 Skin types

Skin type	Tanning ability
Type 1	White skin. Never tans, always burns
Type 2	White skin. Burns initially, tans with difficulty
Type 3	White skin. Tans easily, burns rarely
Type 4	White skin. Never burns, always tans
Type 5	Brown skin (Asian and mongoloid)
Type 6	Black skin (Afro-Caribbean)

2. Make maximum use of shade. The Australians have learnt the value of shade and have run campaigns to plant trees in school playgrounds so that their children can relax and be relatively protected from the sun. Maybe we in this country should follow their example.

3. Dress your children in loose, baggy, close-weave cotton clothes. Oversized T-shirts are particularly appropriate. What should not be worn are skimpy clothes such as sundresses which leave the most vulnerable areas like the shoulders exposed. The shoulders and back of the neck receive a good deal of sun exposure when children are playing, and this is the commonest area for severe sunburn. So, they should be covered where possible.

4. A hat with a wide brim that shades the face and preferably the back and sides of the head should also be worn. A straw boater or sun hat is ideal, but a baseball cap can also provide useful protection.

5. Cover exposed parts of your child's skin with sunscreen. A minimum SPF value of 15 which has UVA and UVB screen should be used. It should not, however, be the main method of protection. It really does come fifth on the list here. It is expensive, requires re-application every 3 hours, and is not fully protective. Waterproof sunblock should be used if your child is swimming. Parts of the body which need extra protection are the nose, cheeks, shoulder tops, and feet.

6. Eyes can also be damaged by excessive sun exposure and should be protected. Sunglasses should have a UV (ultraviolet) filter.

The ICRF also advise outdoor workers to use a sunblock of SPF 15 and to cover up. The Health Education Authority also advise people to use high factor sun screens of at least SPF 15. Their 'sun know how' campaign emphasizes covering up, seeking shade, protecting children, generously applying factor 15 sunscreen, and taking care not to burn.

The best advice to minimize the risk of skin cancer is to spend a minimum of time in the sun, wear light protective clothing (taking care to ensure that the weave of the fabric is not too open), and avoid exposure to the sun during the middle of the day between 11 a.m. and 3 p.m. However, pharmacists know that many of their customers are aiming to get a tan while on holiday. Offering advice about the appropriate use of sunscreens to prevent burning and skin damage is reasonable. Pharmacists should always try to recommend a sunscreen with an SPF of at least 15, especially to those who are travelling to tropical countries. People who are prone to cold sores which may be triggered by UV radiation should be advised to use a lip salve with a high SPF.

Sunscreens with protection against both UVA and UVB rays are needed. Although sunscreens increase the length of time that can be spent in the sun without burning, it should be remembered that this in itself can result in greater overall exposure to the sun. Sunscreens should be reapplied regularly and new supplies bought each year (advise customers to check 'use by' dates).

Targeting advice at parents to prevent or minimize sunburn in their children is important. While adults may be prepared to expose themselves to risk, they may be more likely to respond to advice to protect their children against the future risk of skin cancer. Sun penetrates water, so swimming poses a particular risk of burning. Wearing a shirt protects the shoulders. Both children and adults should be encouraged to wear a hat in the sun.

Advice can also be given on when the sun is strongest and burning most likely. The risk is greater in countries closer to the equator. The midday sun is strongest and sunbathing times should be planned. A simple tip is that when the person's shadow is at its shortest, the sun is overhead and its rays at their strongest. The closer the length of the shadow to the person's actual height, the less strong the sun's rays.

At high altitudes, less of the sun's energy is filtered out, making skin damage more likely and sun protection even more important.

The sun's rays are reflected off snow, so advice about sunscreens for winter holidays is also relevant.

People often prepare for sun protection on hoiday while relatively neglecting it at home. Pharmacists can promote sun protection during sunny weather at home, again emphasizing the importance for children.

14.6   Case studies

1. A man in his 30s asks you for something for diarrhoea.

The pharmacist should routinely ask everyone who presents with diarrhoea if they have recently travelled abroad, along with the other usual questions for responding to symptoms, including the duration. The person should also be asked if there has been any blood in the stools. If they tell you they have been abroad recently, they should be referred to their GP for tests. Antidiarrhoeals may be sold for use until the GP is seen.

2. A woman asks you if it is safe for her 3-year-old son to take antimalarials

All children, even babies, should take antimalarials if they are travelling to endemic areas. Chloroquine is available in syrup form but unfortunately proguanil is not. If the child cannot swallow tablets, parents should be encouraged to crush the proguanil and give it with a spoonful of jam or equivalent to hide its bitter taste. It is very important to explain why continuing the antimalarial after arriving home is necessary. In addition, the pharmacist should tell them that insect repellents and other precautions should always be used.

3. A woman asks for advice about her husband's medication and their forthcoming trip of a lifetime to visit their daughter in Australia. Should he get extra supplies or will he be able to get them while abroad?

It is best to obtain supplies of regular medicines in the UK. In some countries, there may be problems due to poor quality. The potential expense of obtaining them abroad is another issue. It is important not to pack all the medicines in luggage that will be checked in as any delays or lost luggage can then cause problems. Where the person has a recurring condition (for example a woman who is prone to cystitis or thrush), it may be a good idea to take a course of treatment with them in case of supply problems in the holiday country.

References

British National Formulary (current edition)

Daewood, R. (1990) *Travellers' Health: How to Stay Healthy Abroad.* Oxford University Press, Oxford

Department of Health (1998) *Travellers' Guide to Health.* HMSO, London.

15 Drug misuse and harm reduction programmes

Drug misuse includes both licit (prescribed and over-the-counter medicines) and illicit (substances whose use is illegal) agents. Pharmacists come across drug misuse on an everyday basis, and pharmaceutical care of those misusing drugs can raise ethical, legal, and moral issues. The guiding principle is that of minimizing the potential harm from drug misuse, in terms of both individual drug misusers and wider society. Policies of harm reduction in relation to injecting drug users first developed in response to the threat of AIDS and are now widely accepted. The prevalence of hepatitis remains high among injecting drug misusers and could be lowered by further harm reduction measures. There are two main areas for pharmacist involvement—health promotion and enhanced services involving subsitute prescribing (including supervised administration of methadone) and needle exchange. The knowledge base and interpersonal skills of the pharmacist and other pharmacy staff are particularly important in dealing with individuals who are misusing drugs. A non-judgmental and professional approach is essential. Involvement with and an awareness of problem drug users, including registered addicts, are also important. The pharmacist should liaise with local agencies providing services for drug misusers and work closely with them.

15.1   What is drug misuse?

The World Health Organization defines dependence on drugs in this way: 'A person is dependent on a drug or alcohol when it becomes very difficult or even impossible for him/her to stop taking the drug or alcohol without help, after having taken it regularly for some time. Dependence may be physical or psychological, or both'. Another definition is that of the Royal College of Psychiatrists:

'Any taking of a drug which harms or threatens to harm the physical or mental health or social well-being of an individual or other individuals, or of society at large, or which is illegal'. The term 'drug addict' is rarely used now by those working in the field and has been superseded by the concept of drug dependence.

Stereotypes of drug misusers persist—the antisocial, archetypal injecting heroin addict who leads a criminal lifestyle to support their habit, and will shoplift from and be violent towards the staff of any pharmacy attempting to provide a service to them. Pharmacists need to step back from such stereotypes and be aware that the potential for drug misuse and the range of drug misusers is far wider. Some drugs may be used occasionally or even regularly without dependence occurring. Three main categories of drug misuse can be identified:

1. Illicit drug use
2. Misuse of prescription-only medicines
3. Misuse of over-the-counter medicines and other substances which may be purchased legally.

15.2   Illicit drug use

During the twentieth century, the control of drugs which are liable to misuse has become ever tighter in response to wider use in the community. In the nineteenth century, the use of laudanum and other opiates began in the higher social classes and amongst the artistic community (see, for example, Coleridge, and de Quincey in *Confessions of an English opium eater*) and subsequently became widespread. Other famous 'users' were some of the English Pre-Raphaelites, for example the poet and painter Dante Gabriel Rossetti. Concern at the effects of the extensive use of laudanum in society, including its common use in babies and small children to treat a variety of symptoms, led to controls over its distribution and sales.

The first controls over heroin were introduced in 1920, when it was classified under the Dangerous Drugs Act. The origins of substitute prescribing were also in the 1920s, as a recommendation of a major government report in 1926, the *Rolleston Report*.

Drug misuse reduced during the years of the Second World War but, in the post-war era, the recreational use of drugs increased, particularly in the 1960s—another time of experimentation. Some of the reasons for this increase were cheap supplies of drugs such as LSD, cross-cultural factors such as the 'hippie trail to India', the changing social climate, and a small but significant number of prescribers who were prepared to prescribe large quantities of drugs of misuse, notably amphetamine injections.

In response to this misuse of groups of medicines other than opiates, Parliament attempted to control the situation. It is interesting for young pharmacists to note that as recently as 30 years ago, barbiturates commonly were prescribed as hypnotics and were not subject to any restrictions. Amphetamines were widely available for slimming purposes, and benzedrine inhalers could be sold over the counter.

It was only with the introduction and implementation of the 1968 Medicines Act that manufacturers of some over-the-counter products were required to review their formulations. Some commonly sold over-the-counter medicines contained relatively high doses of morphine, often in the form of 'chlorodyne' or tincture of chloroform and morphine.

The 1980s saw large increases in the numbers of individuals dependent on opiates, and in the 1990s the widespread recreational use of 'Ecstasy' (methylene dioxymethylamphetamine or MDMA). The government commissioned the production of guidelines on the treatment of drug dependence in 1984 with the intention of encouraging GPs to treat individuals who were dependent on opioids. The guidelines were revised in 1991 and a further revised edition was published in 1999. The first report by the Advisory Council on the Misuse of Drugs was issued in 1988 and recommended the expansion of treatment services for drug misusers. Community drug teams were set up, and the 1995 White Paper *Tackling Drugs Together* led to the setting up of local Drug Action Teams with a brief for harm reduction programmes. A government Task Force on drug misuse reported in 1996, and included a section on the role of the community pharmacist.

15.2.1 Measuring the extent of drug misuse

A particular feature of legislation in the UK between 1968 and 1997 was the facility for drug addicts to be notified to the Home Office.

The Misuse of Drugs (Notification of and Supply to Addicts) Regulations 1973 required doctors to notify addicts to the Home Office. Drugs for which such notification was required were cocaine, dextromoramide, diamorphine, dipipanone (added to the list in 1985), hydrocodone, hydromorphone, levorphanol, methadone, morphine, opium, oxycodone, pethidine, and phenazocine.

An index of addicts was established to provide statistical information on narcotics abuse but was abolished in 1997. The scheme applied only to Class A drugs and so it excluded, for example, benzodiazepines. Amphetamines were also notably excluded. The index was useful in identifying trends in drug misuse, but its major shortcoming was that it represented only a small proportion of misusers—those who were dependent and had sought medical help. There were 43 400 notified drug misusers in the UK in 1996, an increase from 14 785 in 1989. The 1996 data show that 51 per cent of patients were injecting, and that 70 per cent of the total were dependent on heroin. A national survey of community pharmacies in England and Wales in 1995 showed that about half were involved in dispensing controlled drugs (mainly methadone) for an estimated 30 000 users, compared with less than a quarter of pharmacies and an estimated 7700 users in 1988. Just over one-third were selling injecting equipment (up from 28 per cent in 1988) and almost one in five were providing a needle/syringe exchange service compared with 3 per cent in 1988.

The number of notified addicts did not, of course, register the true number of people who misuse notifiable drugs, which was estimated at between 75 000 and 150 000 in 1986. These figures relate only to notifiable drugs and therefore exclude other drugs such as cannabis and amphetamines. The 1986 estimates were that a further 75 000–150 000 people were users of non-notifiable drugs. Recent surveys on the national prevalence of drug misuse show that at least one in four people will use illicit drugs at some time during their life.

Since the abolition of the index of notified drug misusers, regional drug misuse databases have become the main source of information. These are based on voluntary reporting by doctors who record contacts with patients involving any type of drug misuse. The system will allow better planning of services for drug misusers and feedback to doctors on trends in drug misuse.

However, unlike the previous arrangements, the regional databases are anonymous and do not allow the identification of individuals.

15.2.3   Legal classification of drugs of misuse

In the UK, controlled drugs are categorized into classes A–C (on which penalties are based, with Class A drugs dealt with most severely) and Schedules 1–5, which define the legal requirements for prescribing and supply.

Cannabis is subject to stringent restrictions in law and is the only illicit drug where there has been any significant public support for its use to be decriminalized. Public support for further clinical trials of medical uses of cannabis, for example in multiple sclerosis, is now widespread.

In some countries, for example The Netherlands, cannabis use effectively has been decriminalized in an attempt to separate 'hard' and 'soft' drug use. In the Dutch system, cannabis is sold in coffee houses, which must be registered for that purpose, and who pay tax on sales. Should such outlets be found to also sell 'hard' drugs, their licence is revoked. Thus, possession of cannabis for the individual's own use is not a criminal offence in Holland, but penalties remain for those who sell from other than registered outlets. The programme's philosophy is to reduce demand, and there has been a reduction in cannabis use since its introduction. In 17- and 18 year-olds, usage fell from 10 per cent in 1976 to 6 per cent in 1986. The Dutch experience also appears to show that, by separating the supply of 'soft' and 'hard' drugs, the move from the former to the latter is less likely to occur.

However, there is no definitive evidence that decriminalization or legalization would not result in an increase in drug misuse. Currently there are no moves in the UK to decriminalize any controlled drugs.

Whilst it is relatively easy to place misused medicines under a tight regime of legal control, there is little political will to control some other substances such as alcohol. In addition, there are great practical difficulties in controlling widely available materials such as solvents and aerosols, although the Intoxicating Substances Supply Act 1985 protects the under-16s to some extent in this area.

15.3   The move to harm reduction services

Attitudes towards drug misuse have changed significantly since the 1980s. With the widely recognized risk of transmission of HIV through the sharing of injecting equipment and the use of dirty needles, exchange schemes have been established to provide clean injecting equipment to drug misusers without contravening the Misuse of Drugs Act. The schemes also encourage the return of used needles and syringes for safe disposal. Pharmacists increasingly have been encouraged to participate in the provision of such exchange schemes and to sell or supply needles and syringes to injecting drug users. Prior to the emergence of HIV and AIDS and the evidence on transmission, pharmacists were positively discouraged from selling or supplying needles and syringes to injecting drug users on the grounds that this would encourage, and perhaps even extend, such use. As the custodians of controlled drugs, some pharmacists have found the transition to harm reduction strategies difficult to accept. The next sections in this chapter explain the importance of reducing injecting drug use, the basis of harm reduction, and the reasoning behind its implementation.

15.3.1   The importance of reducing injecting drug use

The reduction of injecting drug use is a key aim of harm reduction programmes. Injecting drug use poses risks for both the individual and wider society (see Box 15.1 below). The most serious of these are the transmission of blood-borne diseases (for example HIV and hepatitis) resulting from shared use of injecting equipment.

Drug users' participation in substitute prescribing programmes with oral methadone is an important component of strategies to reduce their injecting drug use. Where injecting cannot be substituted by oral drugs because the individual does not wish to change, health education about safe injecting techniques is essential. The main issues are summarized in Table 15.1.

15.3.2   Principles of harm reduction

The main treatment programmes for drug misusers were in the past geared towards achieving abstinence from drugs. Such programmes

> # Box. 15.1   Medical complications resulting from injecting drug use
>
> - Transmission of infections (including HIV and hepatitis B and C)
> - Skin problems (cellulitis, necrosis)
> - Septicaemia and endocarditis
> - Respiratory problems (pulmonary embolism, pneumonia)

are appropriate and valuable for drug misusers who are motivated to stop their drug use. The 'Stages of Change' model discussed in Chapter 4 shows why programmes aimed at abstinence will only succeed in a small percentage of cases. Those drug misusers who are at the pre-contemplation or contemplation stages will not be ready to commit to giving up drugs. Trying to make them stop will not work. Having accepted that this is the case, the issue becomes how to minimize potential harm from their drug misuse up to the point where the individual decides they want to try to quit. Harm reduction strategies are based upon this premise, and its principles are shown in Box 15.2 below.

Although the concept of harm reduction has become widely accepted, it is not without its critics. Some (including some pharmacists) argue that harm reduction not only condones but encourages drug misuse. Others claim that the resources used in harm reduction programmes should be used to treat more 'deserving' individuals. It is generally the case that once health professionals understand the principles of harm reduction and the potential drawbacks of not providing such services, they are more likely to accept the concept. This is important, since a network of health professionals, including pharmacists, is essential if harm reduction programmes are to be effective.

Attracting drug misusers to use available services is a key component of harm reduction strategies. It is crucial that the attitude of those involved in providing such services is non-judgemental. Research shows that moralistic attitudes are likely to

Table 15.1　Safer injecting (adapted from *Drug Use and Misuse*, Centre for Pharmacy Postgraduate Education, 1998)

	Key points	Pharmacy issues
The difference between arteries and veins	Recognizing signs that the needle is in an artery rather than a vein	
Injecting paraphernalia and drug preparation	Use of lemon juice, vinegar, citric acid, or ascorbic acid to make heroin soluble	Use ascorbic or citric acid (NB: currently illegal for pharmacists to sell them for this purpose). There is a risk of fungal infection from lemon juice.
	Use of water to dissolve the heroin	Water for injection currently is a prescription-only medicine and cannot legally be supplied
	Use of filters to remove impurities from street heroin	Cotton wool should not be used as a filter—fibres can break off and damage veins
Medical hazards of injecting	Transmission of HIV and hepatitis through shared equipment, and shared use of water for rinsing equipment	Important not only not to share needles/ syringes, but also not to share rinsing water, spoons, and filters
Safer injecting techniques	Use of sterile equipment. If none is available, use of bleach to clean used equipment	Importance of needle/ syringe exchanges or sale of needles and syringes from community pharmacies

deter drug misusers from making or maintaining contact with service providers. Studies with drug misusers themselves show that those using pharmacy services are sensitive to the attitudes of both pharmacists and other pharmacy staff, and that drug misusers will actively seek out pharmacies where they are treated with respect

---

Box 15.2   Principles of harm reduction
(from *Drug Use and Misuse*, Centre for Pharmacy
Postgraduate Education, 1998)

- Provision of accurate information about drug misuse and its risks
- Reaching as many current and potential drug misusers as possible
- Development of the skills of safer drug misuse, e.g. encouraging the oral use of drugs instead of injecting, or if clients are still injecting, encouraging them not to share injecting equipment
- Promotion of more accepting attitudes towards drug misusers

---

and humanity. The role of the pharmacy staff is particularly important here as they often spend much time 'chatting' to drug misusers whilst they are waiting for prescriptions. Some pharmacists have developed written agreements which are signed by both the pharmacist and the drug misuser and set out the service that can be expected and the ground rules for its continuation. Such agreements can reduce unrealistic expectations and clarify the basis of the service (see Wingfield, 1999).

15.3.3   Pharmacy-based harm reduction services

There are two main ways that pharmacists are involved in service provision: supply of drugs via substitute prescribing (for example oral methadone) and syringe/needle exchange schemes. These services are provided in the UK through community pharmacies. Funding is through national arrangements for some aspects (for example the basic dispensing fee for daily supply of oral methadone), supplemented by local arrangements for supervision of methadone administration and for needle/syringe exchange schemes. The rationale for these services in terms of benefits to individual drug misusers and to society is set out in Table 15.2.

Table 15.2. Rationale for pharmacy-based harm reduction services for drug misusers

Service	Benefits to the drug misuser	Benefits to society	Other comments
Substitute prescribing of oral methadone	Reduces risks from injecting drugs. Stabilizes drug intake	Reduction in illicit heroin use. Reduction in drug-related crime (e.g. burglaries)	Brings drug misusers into regular contact with a health care professional
Syringe/needle exchange schemes	Availability of clean, safe needles and syringes. Reduces sharing of needles and syringes	Reduction in transmission of HIV and hepatitis. Reduction in long-term costs of caring for infected patients	Brings drug misusers into regular contact with a health care professional
Supervised administration of oral methadone	Introduces control into drug misusers' often chaotic lives. Promotes accurate dose titration to match to level of addiction	Ensures the individual drug misuser takes their intended treatment. Reduces risk of poisoning children from methadone ingestion. Reduces leakage of methadone onto the illicit drugs market	Brings drug misusers into regular contact with a health care professional.

In addition, pharmacies have an important role in disseminating information about drug misuse, for example through leaflets and participation in local campaigns. The potential levels of involvement of community pharmacists in harm reduction programmes are shown in Box 15.3.

Box 15.3   Potential levels of involvement in harm reduction programmes

Level 1—Display leaflets on drug misuse

Level 2—Provide a dispensing service for substitute prescribing; Sell needles and syringes on request

Level 3—Provide supervised administration of methadone; provide a needle/syringe exchange service; liaise with local drugs agencies and outreach workers; provide talks on drug misuse to local schools; liaise with local prescribers to improve prescribing of drugs liable to misuse

---

15.3.4   Substitute prescribing

Research shows that methadone prescribing programmes reduce illicit heroin use and drug-related crime. Initially, the goal of substitute prescribing was to wean drug misusers gradually off their drugs. Pharmacists and other health professionals sometimes expect the prescribed doses of methadone to reduce. However, a more realistic approach is now taken, and substitute prescribing continues for as long as the individual intends to continue misusing drugs. The 'Stages of Change' model is relevant here (see Chapter 4)—reducing or stopping an individual's supply of substitute drug when they are in the pre-contemplation or contemplation stages is likely to be counter-productive and may lead to restarting of illicit street drugs.

Research has shown that the quality of prescribing of substitute drugs could be significantly improved. Guidelines were issued in 1996, but surveys in 1995 and 1997 showed little change in key areas. There is a role here for pharmacists to liaise with GPs to ensure that the principles of prescribing in this area are fully understood. Good practice includes:

- Daily supply of the drug and, where this is not possible, limiting the quantity prescribed to reduce 'leakage' of excess onto the illicit drugs market

- Use of methadone rather than other opiates
- Use of oral rather than injectable drugs
- Use of liquid rather than tablet formulations
- Supervised self-administration to ensure the dose is consumed and not 'sold on'
- The optimal dose of methadone maintenance treatment is considered to be 50–100 mg daily

Supervised administration of methadone

The 1990s saw the first pharmacy-based schemes where the daily dose of methadone was taken by the individual in the pharmacy under the pharmacist's supervision. These schemes arose from two main concerns. The first was that some individuals were selling their supplies of methadone and thus creating 'leakage' of prescribed methadone onto the illicit drug market. The second was the number of deaths from methadone poisoning among the young children of individuals dependent on drugs. Services for supervised administration of methadone currently are most advanced in Scotland, where Glasgow and Grampian have operated and evaluated schemes for several years. Evaluation of both schemes showed a reduction in methadone-related deaths. Grampian has recently introduced a protocol for the shared care of drug misusers between GPs and community pharmacists.

Supply of injecting equipment from pharmacies

It has always been part of the drug culture that misusers share injecting equipment (their 'works'), generally for practical reasons due to equipment shortage. For first-time injectors, it is likely that someone else's 'works' will have to be borrowed to give the first injection. Traditionally, the sale of injecting equipment by pharmacists was seen as condoning illegal drug use and therefore unethical, and it was in 1986 that the RPSGB changed its policy in this area in recognition of the growing threat from HIV and AIDS. This was followed in 1987 by the first RPSGB guidelines on syringe exchange schemes. It is not surprising that many pharmacists who have been qualified for some time have found the huge shift in attitude and policy difficult to accept. Due to concerns that supplying clean equipment without arranging for disposal might increase health risks from discarded needles and syringes, in 1997 the RPSGB issued a statement which is, in effect, an ethical requirement for pharmacists selling injecting equipment to accept returns of used needles and syringes. This policy may encourage more pharmacists to become involved in exchange schemes. On the other hand, it may stop some of those selling needles from doing so as they may not be prepared to handle used equipment.

Syringe exchange schemes began in the UK in the mid-1980s, and government funding was made available from the late 1980s following a number of local pilot schemes. Community pharmacies are well placed to provide an exchange service because of their accessibility, the availability of the pharmacist, the use of pharmacies regularly for both health- and non-health related reasons by much of the population, and the relatively informal and non-threatening atmosphere of the pharmacy. Pharmacy-based exchange schemes are now widespread, and many provide packs containing:

- injecting equipment
- swabs
- a small sharps bin ('cin bin') to the client
- condoms
- health education leaflets
- contact numbers for local drugs services.

Larger sharps bins are used in the pharmacy to receive used equipment. A logo sticker is generally used in the pharmacy window so that drug misusers know that the service is available without having to go into the pharmacy and ask. Payment for the service is generally through an annual retainer plus a fee per exchange negotiated locally with health authorities/boards. Drug misusers may register to participate in an exchange scheme and may be issued with a unique client number, and/or an identifying item such as a credit-type card or key ring. Most schemes have a monitoring system to track the quantities of equipment supplied and returned.

15.3.5   The need for more pharmacists to be involved

Although the increased number of community pharmacies involved in needle exchange schemes and supervised administration of methadone has been welcomed, there is still a need for more sites. Pharmacists may have concerns about safety and security including needle stick injuries, shoplifting, and violence, and these can be discussed with the local scheme organizer and with other pharmacists taking part. A pharmacist who is thinking about participating in a scheme should:

- Talk to the scheme coordinator to find out what is required
- Talk to other local community pharmacists about their experience of participating
- Consider how the service(s) might be provided from their pharmacy premises
- Discuss the idea with their employer
- Discuss the idea with the pharmacy staff and address their issues and concerns.

Providing services for drug misusers is an important role for community pharmacists and likely to become even more so in the future. The RPSGB's Medicines and Ethics contains detailed information on standards and practices associated with both of these activities.

15.4   Misuse of prescribed medicines

This group of drugs comprises those which are prescription-only medicines and which have a common medicinal use (in contrast to some of those in the previous section, for example cocaine, which is rarely used in medical practice, other than in specialist eye and ear, nose and throat treatments).

Misuse of prescribed medicines can take several forms. Controlled drugs such as morphine may be sought by drug addicts. Whilst doctors, including GPs, are not allowed to prescribe for addiction unless they have a special licence, issued by the Home Office, they are still allowed to prescribe controlled drugs for therapeutic purposes. Drug misusers may persuade a doctor of an urgent need, for example acute pain, or may simply pressurize the doctor to prescribe supplies.

Pharmacists need to be aware of the possibility of drug misuse by other health care personnel and should be alert, for example, to prescribers ordering large quantities of controlled drugs on signed orders, presenting signed orders for such drugs regularly, or regularly collecting supplies of prescribed controlled drugs on behalf of different patients. All of these have occurred in the past and, while they are not common, pharmacists should recognize the need for caution.

Other prescribed medicines which have the potential for dependence include benzodiazepines, to which 15–44 per cent of long-term users become addicted. Concern over the effects of such long-term use led to the issuing of a statement by the Committee on Safety of Medicines which recommends that they should not be prescribed other than for short-term use—normally a maximum period of 4 weeks. The Royal Pharmaceutical Society's Council issued a statement in 1989 encouraging pharmacists to become more involved in counselling patients taking benzodiazepines and in discussions with prescribers.

The legal implications of long-term prescribing of benzodiazepines are yet to be decided, but thousands of patients currently are involved in legal actions. While pharmacists have not yet been involved in such litigation, the suggestion has been made that, by continuing to dispense benzodiazepine prescriptions without question, the pharmacist might be liable. Thus, benzodiazepines set a precedent for the future. The pharmacist can reiterate the doctor's advice that these medicines are valuable for short-term use. However, the pharmacist has a professional duty of care, and where there are known or anticipated side-effects from medium to long-term use these should be acted upon.

15.5   Over-the-counter products

The RPSGB's *Medicines and ethics—a guide for pharmacists* contains a current list of over-the-counter medicines known to be subject to misuse. Liaison with local drugs agencies is a good way to keep in touch with local trends and to be aware of any problems with over-the-counter products. Individuals who are dependent on opiates may try to purchase products containing codeine or morphine, but other ingredients are also misused. The use of diphenhydramine in products for the alleviation of temporary sleep disorders has been controversial, and in 1998 a gel-based product was withdrawn because of concerns (although no evidence) about misuse. There have been other examples in the past where the manufacturers of over-the-counter medicines have responded to concerns about misuse by changing formulations to remove active ingredients known to be misused.

Requests for chemicals intended for use in manufacturing or 'cutting' (extending or diluting) illicit drugs may arise in community pharmacies. Substances involved include ascorbic acid, citric acid, and glucose (used in 'cutting' heroin), sodium bicarbonate (used in 'crack'), hydrogen peroxide (used in the manufacture of 'Ecstasy'), and benzyl methyl ketone (a precursor of amphetamine). The sale of ascorbic acid and citric acid to individual drug misusers for the purpose of injecting drugs is illegal under the Misuse of Drugs Act section 9A, a situation which the RPSGB is lobbying to change so that safer injecting practices can be encouraged.

Working with others in drug misuse

Pharmacists need to network with other local contacts involved in services to drug misusers and these may include the local drug centre, the local health promotion specialist in drug misuse, and the organizer of needle exchange and supervised methadone administration programme.

References

Centre for Pharmacy Postgraduate Education. (1998) Drug Use and Misuse. University of Manchester.

Department of Health. (1996) *The Task Force to Review Services for Drug Misusers*: report of an independent review of drug treatment services in England. HMSO, London.

Matheson, C. (1998) Views of illicit drug users on their treatment and behaviour in Scottish community pharmacies: implications for the harm reduction strategy. *Health Education Journal* 57, 31–41.

Matheson, C et al. (1999) Prescribing and dispensing for drug misusers in primary care: current practice in Scotland. *Family Practice*.

Roberts, K. (1997) Drug misuse. Continuing Education Module. *Pharmacy Magazine* September.

RPSGB *Medicines and ethics   a guide for pharmacists*. Published twice yearly.

RPSGB (1998) Working Group Report on Drug Misuse. *Pharmaceutical Journal* March.

Sheridan, J., Strang, J., Barber, N. and Glanz, A. (1996) Role of community pharmacies in relation to HIV prevention and drug misuse: findings from the 1995 national survey in England and Wales. *British Medical Journal* 313, 272–274.

Strang, J., Sheridan, J. and Barber, N. (1996) Prescribing injectable and oral methadone to opiate addicts: results from the 1995 national postal survey of community pharmacies in England and Wales. *British Medical Journal* 313, 270–272.

Strang, J. and Sheridan, J. (1998) Effect of government recommendations on methadone prescribing in south east England: comparison of 1995 and 1997 surveys. *British Medical Journal* 317, 1489–1490.

Wingfield, J. (1999) Reaching agreement with drug misusers. *Pharmaceutical Journal* 262, 131.

Index

Note: page numbers in *italics* refer to figures and tables